Nutrition for Soccer Players

WHAT TO EAT and DRINK
BEFORE, DURING and AFTER
TRAINING SESSIONS and MATCHES

Π0190237

Library of Congress Cataloging - in - Publication Data

Bonfanti, Mario and Pereni, Angelo
  The Complete Book of SOCCER RESTART PLAYS
      Original title: "CALCIO: Alimentazione e integrazione"

ISBN No. 1-890946-17-6
Library of Congress Catalog card Number 98-067118
Copyright © September 1998
Copyright © Edizioni Correre 1997

First published 1996 by Editoriale Sport Italia Srl Milano Original title: "CALCIO: Alimentazione e integrazione"

Reedswain Books are available at special discounts for bulk purchase. For details, contact Reedswain at 1-800-331-5191.

Editorial coordination
Marco Marchei

Translated from Italian by
Maura Modanesi

Art Direction, Design and Layout
Kimberly N. Bender

Editing and Proofing
Bryan R. Beaver

Printed by
DATA REPRODUCTIONS
Auburn Hills, Michigan

REEDSWAIN BOOKS and VIDEOS
612 Pughtown Road
Spring City, Pennsylvania 19475 USA
1-800-331-5191 • www.reedswain.com

*To those soccer players,
whatever their level,
who believe that
they can always improve
through a proper lifestyle,
through rational training
and through a suitable diet.*

Nutrition for Soccer Players

ENRICO ARCELLI

Published by
REEDSWAIN INC • Pennsylvania

Table of Contents

INTRODUCTION

I n the last few years, many people have gradually come to understand the importance of a proper and well-balanced diet and, for this reason, newspapers and magazines have conformed to modern readers, giving special attention to dietetics. Unfortunately, many of the articles published are not high-quality material: some of them even contain misinformation, while others only raise confusion in the mind of the reader. Lately, I came upon two articles concerning this subject, which appeared in two different magazines almost at the same time. They both dealt with cheese, but in two completely different ways. The first article intended to underline its negative effects on our health, because of its high saturated-fat content; the other one, on the contrary, praised its virtues, in particular the important amount of calcium and noble proteins it offers.

Which was the right article to listen to?

I would say that both the articles were right and wrong at the same time. But, above all, I would add that this conflict of views on the same theme in dietetics brings about two possible considerations. First of all, while speaking of nutrition, it is impossible to exhaust the subject in the few lines of a magazine article: consider for instance the fact that the balance between all the various nutrients is often fundamental in a diet; this is the reason why much more space than a magazine article is needed to explain what this balance really consists of in an exhaustive way, even if the author of the article is a dietitian. Since everyone has a daily relationship with food, there are many who believe that writing about dietetics is a simple matter. Unfortunately, the reader is mainly attracted by the title which not only is made up of few words, but is usually created by a journalist, who necessarily tends to emphasize one particular aspect of the subject.

The second element I would like to underline - and which is partly a consequence of the previous consideration - is the constant spreading of superficial and wrong beliefs about nutrition in modern times. If, for instance, it is true that an excess of bovine meat is not healthy particularly for some persons, it is also wrong to believe that it should be excluded from our diet completely. On one hand, for those who need to lose weight or to digest rapidly, it could be useful to eat one course meals, a dish of pasta for instance, or meat or fish, preceded or followed by cooked or raw vegetables; but on the other hand, this does not mean that this kind of diet is good for everybody, every day at all meals.

Things are even worse when people begin to speak of losing weight. It is true, for instance, that practicing physical activity even for a short time - especially in a hot environment or wearing clothes which do not allow perspiration to evaporate - can help people to reduce their body weight by some pounds; but this is only a loss of water in the form of perspiration and not a loss of fat. We should think of losing weight as losing fat and know that it is fundamental to restore the starting water-balance of our body in order to avoid possible physical disorders. There is also a widespread belief that some kinds of food help people to slim down and therefore can be eaten in large quantities; or that some other kinds of food, eaten at particular hours of the day, do not make people fatten up. Well-grounded and consolidated notions are often completely ignored, while many people embrace ideas born of highly imaginative minds which, unfortunately, do not have the slightest idea of what the foundations of dietetics, and of other sciences, are.

In some cases, computer-based dietology has also helped to muddle people up; for example, some persons occasionally draw up a balance of the nutrients content at every single meal, and according to this balance they judge the whole diet suitable or not, even when this would be senseless, since there are stores of some substances which cannot be burnt up within a few hours. On the contrary, people often forget that eating a large quantity of a particular food, concentrated in one single meal, is different from eating the same quantity divided into many small doses over the course of the day. Suffice to think about table sugar, including highly sugared drinks and food, and the sudden changes in the glycemia and insulin levels which may appear according to whether the sugar intake is broken up into many different moments or not. Moreover, there are some particular substances, amino acids, for instance, which do not accumulate in our body so that, in some specific situations, it would be better to spread their intake out over the various meals of the day, rather than concentrate it in one single meal. Finally, nutrients are usually given too much attention in terms of percentages, thus forgetting something important: our body cannot reason through percentages.

The new sport dietetics

I would say that the difference between the old sport dietetics and the new science of diet and nutrition applied to sport lies in the fact that, in the past, dietetics was mostly based on numbers and focused its attention on particular questions and the relevant answers, such as: How many calories do we need? What is the right amount of carbohydrates? How many milligrams of that specific vitamin does our body need? How long before the performance should an athlete eat?

Today, the old dietology based on numbers has been replaced by a kind of dietetics mainly based on physiological aspects. This does not mean that numbers are no longer important; but before focusing the attention on numbers, it is fundamental to understand how the body of an athlete works while performing physical activity: What are its specific needs? What happens in the body when an athlete eats a particular kind of food or drinks something?

Moreover, according to the old sport dietetics, the diet of sportsmen and women obey the same rules effective for everybody's diet. Most publications on sport dietology, or in the chapters concerning sport in books about general dietetics, still report, for example, that it can help to improve one's sports performance only if there is a deficiency in some particular substances; or that the carbohydrate, protein and lipid content of the diet of an athlete is quite similar to that of sedentary people. But these two considerations are both wrong. Actually, in some cases the sports performance can be improved thanks to suitable diet strategies, even when there is no deficiency at that moment. Moreover, some diets studied expressly for sportsmen are effective just because they are richer or much richer - and in other cases, poorer or much poorer - in carbohydrates, proteins or lipids than the diets suggested to those who do not practice any sport.

I would also add that the origin of the new sport dietetics dates back to a precise moment: the 1969 European track-and-field competition in Athens. During his pre-competition training, Ron Hill, the British athlete who won the marathon, had used a particular food strategy, based on a low carbohydrate diet for some days, followed by a high carbohydrate diet in the days immediately before the competition, which helped him to increase the glycogen level in his muscles. Since then, athletes - including those who do not suffer from any nutrient deficiency - have begun to incorporate other kinds of diet strategies in order to improve their performances; and those strategies were in direct contradiction to the 'rules' valid for sedentary people.

However, sport dietetics has been making considerable progress in the last few years, even though, very often, those who write on this subject have never seen a real athlete, except on TV programs; and even though there are very few sport dietitians who are also in contact with real athletes every day and read scientific journals.

These two reasons, the articles written by incompetent authors and the small number of sport dietitians, are the main factors which still foster the development of diet 'superstitions' among sportsmen. If one sugar lump is good for some athletes in specific conditions, a handful of lumps eaten all together at one single time will undoubtedly have negative effects. Yet, there are people who eat sugar lumps during tennis matches or at halftime of a soccer match. But there are also new 'superstitions' spreading in more recent times.

Carnitine, a substance that our body can synthesize in large quantities and whose function, carrying fatty acid fragments into the mitochondrion, has no particular importance in soccer, a sports discipline where athletes mostly consume carbohydrates, is often considered to be a miraculous element. But, as a matter of fact, it has never helped anybody to improve their own performance.

Dietology applied to soccer

Even though there are still a lot of contradictions underlying this theme, it is possible to state that dietetics has been making considerable progress in the soccer world too. Until only a decade ago, soccer doctors were traumatologists and orthopedists at best; and at that time the attention was mainly focused on injured players. But traumatologists and orthopedists were inevitably hardly acquainted with dietology, a subject which was not investigated during the years necessary to get a medical degree. For this reason, it often happened that players were forbidden to eat pasta, usually referring to the diets used by athletes in the United States or in Great Britain, two countries where pasta was almost unknown at that time, and where it was therefore not recommended to athletes. Today, on the contrary, pasta has been re-introduced into the diet of soccer players for two main reasons: on one hand, there are more experts in sport dietology and, on the other side, throughout the world people know this nutriment and are aware of its importance in the diet of an athlete.

Until some years ago, it could happen that overweight players were advised to drink little and to perspire profusely, just because slimming was erroneously confused with a decrease in the body weight. Now re-plenishing fluids is considered to be fundamental.

In this book

My chief aspiration and purpose while writing this book is to make myself understood by the reader. For many years, I have been following athletes of many different sports disciplines and I have been working with professional soccer teams for a long time. When athletes ask me for help with their nutrition, I do not confine myself, because I have never thought it was the right solution to simply give them a diet table, even a computerized table prescribing 87 grams of one food and 46 grams of another one. Besides, athletes are often obliged to live away from home - even abroad - many days a month and for this reason, it would be senseless to tell them to eat so many grams of one nourishment and so many of the other, since they are unlikely to find particular kinds of food in the place where they are at that moment. I have always followed another way, a longer and more difficult solution, both for them and for me, but undoubtedly safer: I usually persuade athletes to become their own dietitians. In short, I have always tried to improve their knowledge about dietetics, so as to help them to properly choose by themselves what they should eat and drink at every meal of the day, also in case of set choices between unusual foods.

In the world of sport, there are some physicians who act as magicians with the main purpose of developing in their athletes a sort of dependence on them. On the contrary, while speaking to some top-class players, I have often told them that my task was to make myself useless. I am a good dietitian only when I succeed in offering them all the information they need to become self-sufficient in the shortest time possible. In order to achieve this goal as quickly as possible, I have always done my best to try to use a simple language to be understood clearly, as in this book.

In the same way, I have always tried to give top priority to the more common problems that athletes face and have to tackle every day, and at every meal, resorting to theoretical explanations only to help them to better understand the reason why they should choose one particular kind of food rather than another one. For this reason, in these pages I have not followed the ordinary layout of dietology books, which usually start with theoretical information, the calorie balance, the definition of proteins, lipids.... I have immediately begun by suggesting how a player should behave in the most typical situations (match, training, when he is a little overweight and so on) and I have collected the most purely theoretical aspects in the appendices of the book for those who want to further investigate the subject.

Food supplements

The last chapter of this book deals with food supplements. In the last few years, some experts have been firmly opposing the use of these substances in sport, considering them to be 'artificial' elements, in contrast with the 'genuine nature' of food; but, unfortunately, these people do not realize that their position is absolutely anti-historical.

I will immediately explain my assertion. None of any of the foods used by the human being, apart from milk and only in the first months after birth, has been created to be eaten by man. By simplifying the reality, the human being began to use only some of all the substances of both animal and vegetable origin existing in nature: probably berries, roots, worms and the eggs of some birds. Then, with the experience handed down from generation to generation, and many centuries before knowing his real food requirements or before knowing the existence of vitamins, the human being gradually selected other substances present in the environment where he was living.

Step-by-step, man also understood that one single nutriment was not enough, but that it was necessary to combine some different kinds of food. Actually, different nourishments contain different substances combined together: for instance, while eating meat, not only do I ingest the proteins I need, but I also absorb saturated fats which, on the contrary, can be injurious to my health in some cases.

In a sense, the human being has also always eaten different kinds of food because there isn't any complete and perfect nutriment providing, by itself, all the necessary substances, and even when eaten in suitable proportions, and excluding superfluous or noxious elements. Therefore, combining different nourishments, each one with its own flaws, the human being tried to reach a compromise - mainly at an unconscious level - which, without causing him great problems, especially within a short time, provided him with everything he needed to feel well and not fall ill, that is the minimum supply of calories and main nutrients.

In the course of the centuries, man has gradually begun to process the substances he could find in nature in order to obtain those components he needed most. From wheat seeds he got the flour he then used to make very different kinds of food; he used milk to produce cheese, grapes to obtain wine and olives to get oil. Moreover, he cooked nutriments in different ways and processed them so as to improve their preservation; he selected those animal or vegetable species from which he could obtain the best nutriments.

In the last decades, our diet has undergone considerable changes and the knowledge of food and nutritional requirements has improved a lot: people have realized that both the excess and the deficiency of some substances, present in nutriments, can have even long-term effects - positive or negative. This fact has undoubtedly influenced, and will probably affect even more in the future, our priorities when choosing our nourishment. In the meantime, food production techniques have also improved. Today, for instance, table sugar - a 99.6% pure substance - can be produced in large quantities starting from vegetable products (sugar beet or sugar cane). In other words, thanks to the gradual development of dietetics, the human being can now have single substances at his disposal, dissociated from other substances he could not eliminate, but which were often useless or even harmful. This is exactly the case of some elements such as vitamins, minerals and also some food supplements used in sport.

In the next few years, food processing will undoubtedly undergo other important changes and some of them will inevitably affect the athletes' diet.

Even though it may sound paradoxical, according to modern

dietitians a tablet of branched-chain amino acids is more 'natural' for man than a cup of sugared coffee. This is due to the fact that, since his origin, the human being has always used, or better: he has always had to eat branched-chain amino acids, substances which are as fundamental as vitamins. Otherwise he would have fallen ill and died. Sugar, on the contrary, is not necessary for man to survive at all, and neither to feel well; the same is true for coffee which was discovered only a few centuries ago. In Europe it has been used for a little more than 300 years.

1

Diet and Competition

The match represents the most important moment for a player, since it is only during the match that he can test his real value. Therefore, if it is always necessary for him to have a suitable diet, adequate for soccer and to his own individual features, it is also fundamental for him to properly choose what to eat and drink before and during the match - for a better athletic efficiency. Also the post-match diet is important for a player in order to be in the best condition for the following training sessions and also for the following match, particularly when he has to play another competition after only three days or even sooner.

Before the match

Many soccer players at the professional, amateur and youth levels still make serious mistakes with regards to their diet in the hours immediately before a match. Some of these diet errors do not jeopardize the athletic performance purely because athletes - young players in particular - have digestive capacities above the average. For this reason, there can be no physical effects even though, for instance, they eat some kinds of food which are inadvisable by themselves or because they are improperly combined with other nutriments. Other diet errors, on the contrary, are not so venial, since they cause a certain decrease in the efficiency levels, even though the player may be completely unaware of it.

When the period without eating is very long and prolonged

Certainly, eating and drinking can affect negatively the physical characteristics and particularly the mental condition of the player. The psychological aspect is rarely taken into consideration; but, in reality, some particular situations, fast hypoglycemia, reactive hypo-

2

glycemia, and hyperlipidemia, can occur as a consequence of a wrong diet and these conditions, combined with the effects of fatigue, can lead to a considerable deterioration of performance.

If, on one hand, it is proven that the wrong food intake can be harmful, on the other side it is also true that an athlete cannot play a match without having eaten for a long period, for instance since the previous night if he has to play in the morning. Hypoglycemia is one of the consequences of a prolonged period without eating. But in order to better understand the meaning of this word, first of all it is necessary to speak about glycemia.

The term glycemia refers to the concentration of one particular sugar - glucose - in the blood. After complete digestion, a normal person usually contains about one gram of glucose per liter of blood. If the glucose concentration tends to decrease, the liver synthesizes the substance and introduces it into the blood stream, until the normal level is restored.

Actually, the liver contains stores of a complex carbohydrate - glycogen - consisting of interconnected chains of glucose molecules. In case of need, these bonds - thanks to the action of specific enzymes - break down, and glucose molecules separate and move into the blood stream, thus restoring the normal concentration of glucose in the blood.

However, glycogen stores in the liver are restricted and, therefore, they are likely to deplete after many hours without food. So, in this situation, the glucose concentration in the blood gradually decreases, thus leading to hypoglycemia. In this condition, the brain cannot work at optimum levels: actually, brain cells - neurons - do not have their own 'fuel' stores and, therefore, they are obliged to 'suck' glucose from the blood in order to satisfy their energy requirements. When the glucose concentration is lower than the average, that is in the case of hypoglycemia, the flow of this sugar from the blood into the neuron is much more difficult, and, consequently, the neuron itself cannot work at maximum efficiency.

This is the reason why those people who have not eaten for a long period are usually less clear-headed, have slower reflexes and their brain activity is less efficient. Research carried out on junior high school students who had eaten nothing since the night before, have shown that their mid-morning efficiency was very low, without their being aware of this in most cases. According to the results of

THE 10 RULES FOR THE PRE-MATCH MEAL

1. There is no kind of food that, eaten in the hours immediately before the match, allows an athlete to play better.

2. There is, on the contrary, a rational way to eat, which helps players to be much more efficient; and there are also wrong diets which cause a considerable decrease in the efficiency levels.

3. First of all, it is important to eat nutriments which - for their quality and quantity, and also for the way they are combined - can be completely digested in the period between the end of the meal and the beginning of the pre-match warm up.

4. High starch foods (pasta, rice, bread, potatoes....) are easy to digest; they also stimulate the development of glycogen stores in muscles, a substance from which muscles get most of the energy they use during a match. Therefore, at the pre match meal players should prefer starchy nourishments to other kinds of food and they can eat them abundantly.

5. At the pre-match meal, on the contrary, it is useless - or better, it is unadvisable - to eat high protein foods, (different kinds of meat, eggs, cheese...) and, above all, fatty nutriments both the visible ones such as butter, margarine and different kinds of oil, and those fats combined with other substances such as fatty meat, most kinds of cheese, creams and so on.

6. It is important to reduce the intake of simple sugars, that is to say the intake of highly sugared foods and drinks, starting from common table sugar, or sucrose, and glucose, or dextrose.

7. For an easy and rapid digestion, it is fundamental to focus the attention on the combination of nutriments; for instance, it would be better not to eat fruit at the end of the meal, or not to eat two different kinds of high protein foods, such as meat and cheese, meat and eggs, eggs and cheese, milk and meat, milk and eggs... In case of a morning match, white coffee should be avoided.

8. In order to help digestion, it is possible to have a one-course meal, that is to say one main course, particularly abundant, preceded or followed by a dish of fresh or cooked vegetables.

9. When the match is going to be played in particular environmental conditions, which will cause players to perspire profusely (sunny weather, high temperature and humid), it is advisable not to drink alcohol in the 24 hours preceding the competition.

10. When it is possible to foresee that players will perspire profusely during the match, it is worthwhile drinking two glasses of water, pure or added with suitable salts, just before entering the playing field.

scientific research, typists and precision workers are also more likely to make mistakes if they have eaten nothing since the previous night.

Blood glucose concentrations lower than the average negatively affect not only our mental efficiency, but also our physical condition. For these reasons, a player should never play a match if he has not eaten anything within the previous eight hours.

When there is little glycogen in our muscles

Glycogen is present also in our muscles; but, once they have broken down, glucose molecules cannot leave this area: they are used by our muscles - and only by them - as fuel. During hard muscular work, long training, a very exhausting practice, or a match, there is little glycogen left in our muscles; as a consequence, they are less efficient and, from the physical point of view, the performance itself is affected negatively. In order to re-plenish glycogen stores in our muscles, it is necessary to absorb carbohydrates, for instance by eating bread, pasta, rice, fruit and so on. One of the main purposes of the pre-match diet is the possibility to increase the glycogen concentration in muscles, even though - to tell the truth - it can be raised to the highest levels only through a suitable diet protracted for many hours, or even some days, as you can read below, in the section 'After the match'.

When the digestion is still taking place

As I said before, a protracted period without food is a real dietetic error; but it is also possible to make the opposite mistake: finishing one's meal a short time before the beginning of match. If the period between the end of the meal and the beginning of the pre-match warm up is excessively short, and/or the player has eaten wrong foods, or even combined improperly, some gastric disorders, (something lying heavy on the stomach, acidity, nausea, vomiting), or some general problems (dizziness, feeling weak) may appear while the player is on the field because his digestion is not finished yet. There is a mutual influence - which is particularly harmful for the performance - between digestion and physical activity when they both occur at the same time: actually, each one of these two processes affects the other in a negative way. Also our brain often experiences negative effects when food still lies heavy in our stomach.

Therefore, which are the nutrients to exclude from or to prefer for the pre-match meal? Here are, in detail, some suggestions.

Very few fats - The first rule to observe for an easier digestion is reducing the fat content in the meal preceding the match. In particular, it is necessary to avoid fried food and fats cooked a long time. It is fundamental to exclude fatty meat. In the same way, it is important to remove particularly fatty parts from meat, the skin of the chicken and so on. It is unadvisable to eat those parts of the roasts or of roast beef in direct contact with cooking fats. Sauces, condiments, cheese, and whole milk should be reduced. As for real fats (butter, margarine, different kinds of oil...) it is necessary to use them in very small quantities and preferably raw. Fats require a very long time to be digested completely and also prolong the digestion period of the other nourishments they are eaten with. Even once they have been digested and they finally arrive into the blood, they are a nuisance: actually, hyperlipidemia, the excess of lipids or lipid-like substances in the blood, which appears in case of a high fat diet, impairs the efficiency of the brain.

Few proteins - It is not necessary to eat proteins at the pre-match meal, so it is possible to abstain completely from high protein nourishments, such as different kinds of meat, eggs, cheese milk... But some players feel a sort of psychological need to absorb these foods. In these cases, it is advisable to eat - as I have already said before - some slices of, or a small portion of, very lean meat cooked without fats.

Complex carbohydrates in abundance - High carbohydrate nutriments are usually the easiest to digest and they also stimulate the development of glycogen stores in our muscles and in the liver. It would be better to eat complex carbohydrates, polysaccharides, and starches, such as those contained in pasta, bread, rice, potatoes and so on.

Avoid ingesting too much simple sugar - It is important to reduce the ingestion of simple carbohydrates (monosaccharides), that is simple sugars like sucrose - the common table sugar - and glucose, also known as dextrose. When these sugars are ingested in too large a quantity and at one single time, the glucose concentration in the blood rapidly increases, (hyperglycemia). Then, insulin, a protein hormone secreted in the pancreas, is released into the blood in much higher amounts than the average.

Therefore, glycemia is brought back to normal levels; but - if the glucose rate and, consequently, the insulin concentration grow considerably and too rapidly - it may also happen that glycemia drops under normal levels. This condition is known as reactive hypoglycemia, a sudden deficiency of sugar in the blood as a response to the excessive glycemia increase, see the box on page 7 and the diagram it contains.

As I said before, hypoglycemia promptly impairs the efficiency of the brain; for this reason, it is advisable for a player to consume only the minimum amount of drinks and food particularly rich in sucrose (table sugar), or glucose. In reality, some starchy nourishments also tend to raise glycemia levels, and, consequently, insulinemia levels too: but, this does not happen so suddenly as in the case of these two sugars.

Avoid wrong combinations, taking a one-course meal if necessary. As I will explain in the section '**Food combinations**' on page 56, it is very common to combine two different nutriments which necessarily require two different digestive processes. This often causes disorders. For this, we should avoid eating fruit at the end of our meal when we want to have a more rapid digestion. Also, combining starchy food (pasta or rice), with protein (steak or other kinds of meat, eggs, cheese...) requires longer digestion times than those needed to digest only one course. The same is also true when combining two proteins, meat and cheese, meat and eggs, eggs and cheese, milk and meat, milk and eggs.

In the last few years, many soccer players have gradually grown accustomed to having exclusively one-course meals - above all at midday, especially if there is a training session in the afternoon. It consists of a generous portion of one main course (pasta or rice, or, more rarely, meat or fish) followed or preceded by a dish of cooked or, still better, fresh vegetables. In this way, the digestion period is generally shorter than the time needed to digest a two-course meal.

How Sugar Intake and Ingestion
Can Cause Reactive Hypoglycemia

When sucrose (common table sugar) is ingested at one single time in a quantity equivalent to several teaspoonfuls, some unpleasant consequences may occur in our body, particularly for those who, like soccer players, have to perform physically (training or match) within a short time.

Sucrose is a disaccharide, a sugar consisting of two linked monosaccharide molecules or simple sugars: one molecule of glucose and a fructose molecule; when sucrose gets into the digestive tube, the two elementary molecules split up and are absorbed separately. Contrary to what we could think, these two operations, splitting and absorption, take place in a very short time, particularly if sugar has been ingested on an empty stomach and if it is dissolved in a drink.

While fructose, at least in small doses does not create any problem, glucose - when it is absorbed and released into the blood - causes an increase in the glycemia levels, the word glycemia exactly refers to the glucose concentration in the blood.

Every time glycemia rises, that is in case of hyperglycemia, there is also a consequent reply by the body, and by the pancreas in particular. Insulin is released into the blood in a higher quantity than the average amount for a hormone.

If glycemia has increased abruptly, for instance because the person in question drank a can of soda containing ten grams of sugar on an empty stomach, the blood insulin concentration is very likely to grow causing hyperinsulinemia. In this condition, the glucose present in the blood easily flows into the cells - particularly into the cells of muscle fibers and the liver (hepatocytes) and fat (adipocytes): in practice, glucose flows in the blood.

At this point, the blood glucose concentration, glycemia, gradually drops and it can even reach lower levels than the average, which means hypoglycemia, or deficiency of sugar in the blood. This kind of hypoglycemia is known as 'reactive hypoglycemia', because it appears as a reaction to the previous increase in the glycemia levels.

Nutritionists also speak of a 'rebound effect', since, in a very short time, glycemia suddenly shifts from normal levels to high rates, which, in turn, cause the blood glucose concentration to drop below the average.

It is important to observe that fructose - when it is ingested alone - does not stimulate reactive hypoglycemia, as you can see in the diagram; actually, it is absorbed much more slowly by our intestine.

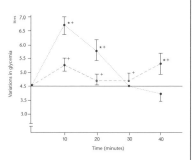

Variations in glycemia, the blood glucose concentration, following the ingestion of glucose, dotted line, fructose, sketched line, or placebo, straight line. In the first case, glycemia rises much more quickly and suddenly drops below basal rates within a very short time, reactive hypoglycemia; on the contrary, the same quantity of fructose causes glycemia to increase much more moderately and does not bring about any fall below average levels.

Some examples of pre-match diets

Considering that a match can be played at different times of the day, it is possible to suggest the following:

Match played in the middle of the afternoon - It is possible to suggest two different kinds of meal which should be eaten two and a half or three hours before the beginning of the pre-match warm up: an Italian style meal and a one-course meal. The latter is the best solution for those players who commonly have digestion problems.

Example A: Italian-style meal
- main course: pasta, or rice, with extra virgin olive oil or butter, or tomato and basil;
- boiled potatoes with little oil;
- a small portion of chicken, cooked without fats;
- a piece of cake;
- one roll, mineral water, either aerated or not, as much as you like, one cup of coffee for those who are accustomed to it.

Example B: one-course meal
- main course: as above, but you can also have a double portion;
- mixed vegetables, cooked or preferably fresh, with a little oil dressing.

Match played in the morning - Drinking coffee with cream is a real mistake which should be avoided; it takes a long time to be digested, especially in conditions of stress - and players are often unaware of the stress which exists before every competition, even the less important ones. Coffee with cream can cause gastric acidity, the sensation of something lying heavy in the stomach, and, sometimes, nausea, vomiting and headache.

In order to avoid these problems, it is advisable to follow these suggestions:
- bread with a thin layer of honey or marmalade (it is better to avoid butter);
- cookies are often difficult to digest;
- tea, coffee or milk.

9

Match played in the very early afternoon - During the winter season, matches usually begin in the very early afternoon. There are some players who have to leave home in the middle of the morning to arrive at the playing field in time for the match. In order to leave a certain interval between the end of the meal and the beginning of the journey, and this interval is particularly important if the player travels by car and has to drive, a player can choose between two different solutions: he can have his breakfast early in the morning and a light lunch (a one-course meal consisting of carbohydrates) just before leaving home or he can have a much richer breakfast than usual later in the morning. In short, he can follow one of these two diets:

Diet A:
• breakfast early in the morning: tea, coffee or milk with bread with honey or marmalade;
• lunch, light: pasta, or rice, with oil or butter, or tomato and basil;
• a dish of vegetables.

Diet B:
• rich breakfast in the middle of the morning: tea or coffee with bread and honey or marmalade;
• one yogurt; a piece of cake;
• one or two fresh fruits or bread with marmalade or honey an hour and a half to two hours before the match.

Match played at night - In the summer period in particular, some matches are played late in the afternoon or at night. In these cases it is better to avoid eating the evening dinner, and it is advisable to have a midday meal rich in carbohydrates and to take a mid-afternoon snack two hours or more before the beginning of the pre-match warm up:
• snack with tea, (bread and honey, a piece of marmalade cake);
• or fresh fruit.

The quick pre-match meal at home or on the road

While college and professional players eat the last meal before the match together, usually in a dining hall or restaurant, most players eat at home, especially if the match is played near where they live. It sometimes happens that some of these players have to eat very quickly before they leave or even on their way to the ground.

What should they choose in this case?
First of all, it is important for the player to eat quite abundantly at the previous meal. For instance, it is advisable to have a rich breakfast if the match is played in the afternoon. Then, considering what was explained above, nutritionists usually suggest eating a little just before leaving, for instance:
• one sandwich, preferably with lean meat;
• a piece of cake and tea.

Immediately before the match

In the past, dietitians used to speak of waiting ration, referring to what was eaten between the last main meal, taken three hours before the match, and the beginning of the competition, that is in the short time preceding the match. Today, nutritionists are inclined to think that players should eat or drink nothing but water with added sugars and salts. Both these substances must be properly dissolved, as you will read below, particularly after warm up and before the starting whistle. In the winter period, a little can be enough, while in summer it is necessary to drink two glasses at least.

There are two exceptions to take into consideration: the first one concerns carbohydrates for those who - for different reasons - haven't eaten anything for six or seven hours. The second exception regards fluids, especially when players know that they are going to play in very difficult weather conditions and, for this reason, they are going to perspire profusely because of high temperature, humidity and very sunny weather.

In the first case, it is useful for a player to ingest nutriments having these two characteristics: they must be easy to digest and they should not cause any sudden variation in the glycemia. As was explained above, when a sugar causes glycemia to rise abruptly, a large quantity of insulin is very likely to be released in the blood, thus leading to reactive hypoglycemia. Therefore, for the first reason it is better to choose simple sugars or maltodextrins; and for the second one, it is advisable to exclude glucose and sucrose,

11

especially if the quantity exceeds tens grams, and to prefer fructose, the sugar that does not bring about reactive hypoglycemia.

With regard to the measures to take when the player knows that he is going to perspire profusely during his match, we refer to the third chapter, which is completely focused on the importance of fluids for soccer players. Now, we only want to underline that the loss of considerable amounts of water (dehydration) and salts by our body impairs our physical efficiency, causes cramp and sometimes can even damage the efficiency of our brain, as a consequence of the increase in the body temperature.

In order to avoid these unpleasant disorders, players should have a pre-hydration, which means that they should drink a lot just before entering the playing field, that is after their warm up. Moreover, if the match is played in extreme weather conditions, players could even consider the possibility to make a pre-hydration consisting of glycerin dissolved in water.

DURING THE SOCCER MATCH

For many years, players have been drinking at half time; but, much more recently, they have begun to drink also during the match, in particular when weather conditions call for it. Only in the last few years have nutritionists started to underline the importance of water and also energy supply in the course of the match.

The importance of drinking during the match

We have already mentioned in the previous paragraph, and we will explain in detail in the second chapter, that the loss of considerable quantities of water and salts in the form of perspiration can seriously affect athletic efficiency. For this reason, players should try to replenish most of the lost substances. So, besides drinking before the beginning of the match, they should also drink abundantly at half time. Pure water may not be enough. It would be better to add suitable salts or to drink substances expressly marketed for athletes such as Gatorade. The water or the drink can be cooled, but not iced. In the winter season, it is usually sufficient to drink small quantities of fluids, but in extreme weather conditions, which cause players to perspire profusely, it is worthwhile drinking a couple of glasses, starting immediately after the end of the first half. In other words, the trainer or manager should prepare different water bottles in

THE 10 RULES FOR RE-PLENISHING FLUIDS DURING THE MATCH

1. During the match, the player may need to re-plenish water, added with salts, if necessary, and energy, in the form of carbohydrates.

2. The quantity of water a player should drink during a match varies according to weather conditions; it is also important to decide the amount of salts to dissolve in water.

3. When the match is played in cold weather conditions, it is sufficient for a player to drink only after the warm up and at half time.

4. The higher the temperature, humidity, and sun radiation levels are, the greater the quantity of fluids a player should drink.

5. When the match is played in extreme weather conditions, causing players to perspire profusely, the drink should also contain a certain amount of salts.

6. In these conditions, besides drinking after the warm up and at half time, players should drink also during the match, whenever they can get an opportunity.

7. In case of extreme weather conditions - exceptional temperature, high humidity, and sun radiation - players should consider making a pre-hydration, that is drinking water added with glycerin 60 to 90 minutes before the beginning of the competition.

8. With regard to energy supply, players should re-plenish carbohydrates, which means ingesting simple sugars, fructose, glucose, sucrose, and/or maltodextrins.

9. For those players who have a normal glycogen concentration in their muscles before the match, it is probably sufficient to drink fluids containing carbohydrates immediately before the competition and at half time.

10. Those players who usually run a lot should drink carbohydrates more than once in the course of the match, even in winter, when drinking small quantities of water would normally be enough.

advance, and give them to the players as soon as the referee whistles for the interval. The players should drink - if they can - also during the match, particularly during the pauses caused by injuries. When it is hot, the trainer or manager usually carries one or more water bottles, containing sugars and salts dissolved in water, when entering the field, so the players can easily get one of these or run to the bench to drink. It is better to drink a little every time, or, when players are perspiring profusely, they can drink the maximum quantity of fluids which, according to their experience, can be ingested easily without causing them any problem. In very humid environmental conditions it is possible to produce a much higher amount of perspiration per minute than the water supply which - even in ideal conditions - can be restored by drinking. For this reason, the first 45 minutes can be enough to lead to a considerable dehydration rate.

The importance of re-plenishing energy during the match

While referring to soccer, people are usually prone to think that water - or, If necessary, water added wIth mIneral salts - Is the only element which can gradually deplete and must be re-plenished during a match. Even though, in the past, soccer players were traditionally given a cup of sugared tea at half time, sugar, as well as lemon, were added above all to enhance its taste.

But, in 1992, A. Sassi and L. Somenzini started to point out the importance and the benefit of also re-plenishing energy in the course of a soccer competition.

However, at the end of the sixties, through muscle biopsies (diagnosis by removing small fragments of muscle tissue for examination), carried out on players belonging to the best Swedish clubs, Karlsson, (see the diagram in the box on page 15) had observed that the muscle glycogen concentration rapidly dropped during the first half and got minimum or practically zero levels at the end of the match. It is fundamental to remember that in soccer, muscles get the energy to work mainly from glycogen. For this reason, those players who had little glycogen in their muscles usually ran less than the others.

According to O'Brien and his colleagues (1993) a player can spend about 425 grams of glycogen during a match, 325 of them provided by his muscles and 100 by the liver. When the whole of this glycogen is used in the aerobic mechanism (a process in which glycogen combines with oxygen to provide energy) it produces about 1900 calories.

It is also important to note that no soccer player, not even the most efficient one, can spend so much in the course of the whole match (Arcelli and Ferretti, 1993). However, glycogen is completely, or mostly, consumed in the lactic acid-based energy mechanism, a process helping lactic acid to build up in muscle fibers, (Arcelli, 1995). This process implies carbohydrate consumption and, as a consequence, it causes glycogen stores to deplete much more rapidly than in aerobic mechanisms providing the same amount of energy.

According to Sassi and Somenzini (1992) soccer players should always ingest drinks containing carbohydrates - for instance, fructose and maltodextrins - in concentration equal to or lower than 5% during the match. Actually, carbohydrates would prevent hypoglycemia, that is the decrease in glycemia below normal levels. Hypoglycemia has been discovered in some soccer players at the end of a match. However, to tell the truth, it does not appear in all players, but only in a small percentage. Those who suffer from this deficiency tend to feel very weak and to have slower reflexes, so that these particular conditions cannot ensure a good performance during the competition.

GLYCOGEN IN MUSCLES AND ITS DEPLETION DURING THE MATCH

The muscles of soccer players draw the energy they need to work above all from the carbohydrates present in muscles and in the liver in the form of glycogen. In order to imagine what glycogen really is, you can think of a very small ball made with the soft inner part of a loaf of bread; now, think of reducing it many thousands of times. Well: a great number of these extremely small sodden balls can be found in muscle fibers, but also in liver cells. Glycogen, as well as starch, the main substance occurring in the soft inner part of bread, consists of a very high number of glucose molecules, connected one to the other. When one molecule is needed, it is cut off the chain and used.

The diagram below shows that soccer players usually use up almost all the muscle glycogen stores within the 90 minutes of a competition; however, some of them start the match with low glycogen stores in their muscles, that is less than one gram per a hundred grams of muscle tissue. So, these players spend nearly all the glycogen by the end of the first half. It is important to underline that the total depletion of muscle glycogen stores, or its depletion in most fibers, seriously impairs the physical efficiency of players.

Getting used to practicing aerobic training and having a diet rich in carbohydrates at the meals preceding the match, or even in the last three or four days - choosing foods according to the suggestions in the table on page 21 - can help players to raise their muscle glycogen concentration. Actually, this concentration can rise from 1.4-1.8 grams of glycogen per one hundred grams of muscle tissue - the typical levels of a sedentary person having a mixed diet - to considerably higher rates, even more than doubled. This is probably the reason why a much more recent research by Shephard and Leatt (1987) shows higher levels of muscle glycogen at the beginning of the match, and smaller reductions after the competition, compared to the figures in the diagram, by Karlsson (1969).

On the contrary, those players who have a diet poor in carbohydrates at the meals following a match or strenuous exercise, risk facing the following competition with low glycogen stores; this is exactly what happened to two of the players considered in the diagram. Many athletes are persuaded that eating low carbohydrate meals can help them to lose weight. But - especially when two matches are played within a short time - this can cause their muscle glycogen concentration to be very low when they begin the second competition. Therefore, their athletic efficiency is impaired, particularly at the end of the first half and during the second one.

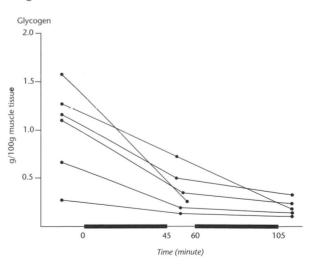

Muscle glycogen concentration, grams per one hundred grams of fresh muscle tissue, prior to the beginning of a soccer match in the Swedish first division, at half time and after the competition. From Karlsson (1969) then revived by Ekblom (1986) and finally modified.

Moreover, the carbohydrates ingested during the match can provide muscles with an energy supply, which is particularly important when the muscle glycogen concentration is very low. Practically, muscle fibers lacking glycogen can keep on working, using the energy provided by ingested carbohydrates.

The carbohydrate intake during the match is beneficial especially to those players who - because of a wrong diet, for example - face the match having a low glycogen concentration in their muscles. However, in these cases it would be more reasonable to advise them to eat in a much more rational way on the day of the match and on the days preceding the competition! But, in my opinion, it can be profitable also for those athletes who have performed strenuous exercise during the match and, therefore, have used up a larger amount of glycogen.

The better athletic efficiency soccer players have been acquiring in the last few years inevitably results in a greater need for integration: as a matter of fact, water and salts integration is fundamental because - in equal environmental conditions - those who run more than others in the course of the match inevitably produce more metabolic heat and, therefore, usually tend to perspire more profusely. But also energy integration plays an important role, since glycogen consumption tends to grow during the match, even though muscle glycogen concentration usually rises in those players who train everyday. The depletion of glycogen stores affects an increasing number of fibers so that it is extremely useful for a player to re-plenish carbohydrates while playing a match.

For these reasons, those who usually run a lot should take a drink containing carbohydrates providing energy, with fructose and maltodextrins, for instance, not only at half time, but also during the match - twice a half, for example, obviously according to the pauses in the play. These 'quick supplies' should be experimented with during training sessions and friendly matches or matches preparing for important competitions; they should consist of 100 grams of drink and at least 5 grams of carbohydrates every time, provided that these substances have a 5% concentration. Every player should gradually understand - after his experiences during training sessions or friendly games - which is the maximum amount of fluids he can drink without any serious disorder appearing.

Today, soccer players often ingest drinks containing not only salts, but also carbohydrates, in particular when it is terribly hot, or the humidity and sun radiation levels are very high, and, therefore, they are very likely to perspire profusely. Athletes should resort to fluid and energy integration in a much more systematic way, including when the climatic conditions do not cause players to perspire abundantly, as in the winter period.

AFTER THE MATCH

I do not like appearing as a person who always wants to say the contrary of what others say, but I am completely persuaded that a lot of people tend to make some mistakes regarding the post-match diet. Unlike in the past, in the last few years we no longer hear people assert that players can neither drink nor eat in the hours immediately after the match. Those who were in favor of the post-match fast stated that the body was exhausted because of the effort of the performance and that it had to partly recover its original condition before making another effort for digestion. First of all, those persons did not understand that the organs involved in these activities are different, the organs of the locomotor apparatus on one side, and those of the digestive system on the other, and that it is therefore senseless to believe that there is an addition of efforts. Moreover, they did not realize that drinking and eating can help players to recover more rapidly from some of the components of the stress caused by the competition.

However, if it is true that players are no longer told not to drink and eat in the hours immediately after the match, it is also true that some people insist upon diets leaving very few choices, extremely punitive and not particularly beneficial for players from a practical point of view.

Why players can lose their appetite, but not their thirst....,

It is true that some players have no appetite immediately after the match. Actually, the effort of the performance triggers the production of catecholamines, endorphins and other hormones in the blood, causing hunger to disappear completely. This is a factor which could be considered as a sign of the fatigue of the body as a whole, and I believe there is no reason for ignoring it. In other words, a player should not make the effort of eating if he does not want to. It is much more important for players to drink and to choose suitable drinks providing at least ten grams of sugar - especially if they have to play another match within two or three days, as will be explained in the following pages.

However, almost all players are thirsty at the end of a match and their thirst rises according to the perspiration they produced during the performance and, to air temperature, humidity, and sun radiation. In my opinion, it is important to begin drinking immediately after the end of the match. It is better to drink a little, but quite often, preferably sports drinks to pure water (see chapter 3). As a matter of fact, it takes a very long time to re-plenish water, it can even take some hours when the player has lost more than 3 liters of fluids, and a dehydrated person, lacking salts, is more vulnerable to different kinds of problems.

The snack and the dinner after the match

If the match ends in the middle of the afternoon, players can have a snack a short time later: for instance, they can eat foods like bread with marmalade or honey; cookies; apple pie or other cakes; fresh fruit - and drink something like tea or a fruit-shake.

At the evening dinner, it is top priority to ingest a lot of carbohydrates, few proteins and very few fats. The reason for this suggestion will be further investigated in the following paragraph and in the box on page 22. Therefore, players should prefer pasta or rice, even in generous portions, but with few condiments and sauces while fried fats or fats cooked for a long time must be avoided. Meat, eggs, cheese... can be restricted to small portions, while fresh or cooked vegetables should not be excluded; also a dessert is permitted (fruit ice cream, cakes without cream or custard). It is important to drink water or citrus fruit juices or fruit shakes in order to quench one's thirst.

Re-integrating glycogen

In case of two matches played a few days apart, or even on two days running, as it happens during some tournaments, it is fundamental for players to follow specific elementary rules not only at the main meals between the two competitions, but also in the minutes immediately after the first match. Only if players completely understand these rules can they be certain to bring their glycogen stores back to normal levels and not to face the second match with those deficiencies which would inevitably reduce their abilities and impair their performance.

As I have already stated, at the end of a soccer match the muscles of a player have used up most glycogen, or the whole of it, that is that kind of starch from which muscle fibers draw most of the energy they use to work. Notice that it takes a longer time to restore glycogen than to re-plenish water. In fact, it can take up to ten hours. Moreover, it is essential to consider that water re-plenishing is stimulated by thirst, urging athletes to drink, and, consequently, to introduce water. Restoring glycogen stores is much more complex. As a matter of fact, if players trust their subjective sensations exclusively and do not choose the right nutriments in a rational way, their glycogen stores are likely to be still nearly depleted after some days. As we said before, this condition inevitably impairs the athletic performance of players and this is particularly dangerous when they are going to play a match, in a cup contest for instance.

Some dietitians suggest that players should ingest ten grams of sucrose (table sugar) immediately after the match via the use of specially made drinks for athletes.

On the contrary, I usually propose to drink - as soon as the referee whistles the final signal and even before taking a shower - two cans of those sweet and carbonated soft beverages, which are absolutely not fit for athletes, with the sole exception of this occasion. It is better to avoid cola drinks, which are usually rich in caffeine, a substance that does not help glycogen reconstruction at all, and to prefer orange or lemon flavored soda. Two cans of these soft drinks contain about 80 grams of table sugar in all, the perfect quantity to start glycogen reconstruction, and athletes usually drink them with pleasure at the end of an effort.

Nearly two hours later, it is useful for players to drink another two cans of soda. Then, at the evening dinner, they should eat above all foods rich in carbohydrates, such as pasta, rice, potatoes and fruit and desserts, excluding those containing cream or custard.

If athletes do respect this scheme, two cans + two cans + starchy dinner, they can restore their glycogen stores at higher levels than they would do if they followed a mixed diet.

If players do not have the suitable glycogen concentration in their muscles, they can be very inefficient and particularly fatigued

THE 10 RULES FOR A RAPID RE-PLENISHING AFTER THE MATCH

1. It is important to recover from the stress of the match in the shortest time possible if another match is going to be played a few days later, midweek for instance, after the Saturday or Sunday competition. It is important also to face the first training session after the competition in the best physical condition.
2. It is fundamental to re-plenish above all water, salts and muscle glycogen after a competition.
3. Water can be re-plenished in different ways: drinking pure water or soft drinks, or eating vegetables, fruit, soups and other nutriments rich in water.
4. A lot of foods help players to re-plenish salts they lost while perspiring. However, a certain nourishment can obviously be rich in a particular kind of salt lost in small quantities and poor in another kind of salt lost abundantly. Those drinks produced especially for athletes, only those with the suitable formula, ensure that players re-plenish all the salts they lost, in the right proportions. In short, the higher the quantity of water evaporated in the form of perspiration, the higher the risk that foods or drinks ingested do not provide the suitable quantity and proportion of salts the body needs.
5. Restoring normal glycogen stores in muscles is possible by eating foods rich in carbohydrates; therefore, the meals preceding and following the competition or the training session must provide a suitable portion of nutriments rich in carbohydrates, such as bread, pasta, rice, potatoes, cookies or other candy, fresh fruit and so on.
6. None of the main meals can consist mostly of foods rich in proteins, unlike those who have a 'dissociated diet' usually do.
7. The sooner the next competition or training session, the earlier a player should begin to ingest carbohydrates and the greater the quantity of carbohydrates ingested during a whole day.
8. If another match is going to be played two days later, it is useful to ingest approximately ten grams of table sugar, (sucrose) immediately after the first match, for instance drinking two cans of a soft drink. The same thing should be repeated two hours later.
9. In order to recover more quickly after the match, it could be useful to ingest branched chain amino acids; in this case too, it is better to ingest them immediately after the competition.
10. If there is no midweek match to play and if players usually feel good at the first training session of the week, they can avoid ingesting branched chain amino acids and they can also follow these suggestions less strictly.

during the training session two days after the match. I do not believe that they should resort to high sucrose drinks, but I suggest that the main meals following the competition, starting from the evening dinner, if the match was played in the afternoon, should be rich in carbohydrates, such as bread, pasta, rice, fruit, potatoes and vegetables, for instance, see the box below.

The most suitable foods and drinks for the snack or the dinner after the match, so as to help rapid glycogen re-plenishing in muscles:

- pasta, rice;
- bread, bread sticks, crackers;
- cookies and candy;
- greens and vegetables;
- all kinds of fruit, excluding oily fruit: walnuts, almonds, hazelnuts, peanuts;
- honey, marmalade, sugar, soda, fruit shakes.

HOW TO RE-CONSTRUCT GLYCOGEN RAPIDLY

Fructose, a common sugar occurring in different kinds of fruit, is undoubtedly advisable in various sports situations; but it is not particularly suitable when the main goal is to re-construct muscle glycogen in the shortest time possible, especially when two matches are played a few days apart, three or less. In these cases, it is better to ingest glucose, also known as dextrose, but also sucrose (table sugar).

While the latter was given great importance in the past, (in some sports disciplines, there were athletes who used to ingest a handful of sugar lumps as soon as they felt their physical efficiency was sinking) in the last few years particular attention has been turned to its disadvantages. In fact, its quick flowing in the blood stream was generally considered as one of its main virtues, while, on the contrary, it is the main flaw of this sugar, and of glucose as well, in most sports situations. The sudden increase in glycemia levels causes plasma insulin concentration, a protein hormone, secreted in the pancreas, to rise quickly; this causes glycemia to drop considerably within a very short time, especially if sugar was ingested in abundant quantities all at once. Hypoglycemia obviously impairs the athletic efficiency of a player, both from the muscle and the mental point of view.

However, for some years, and particularly after the studies carried out by important researchers such as Costill and his colleagues, 1981, Blom and coll., 1987, Ivy and coll., 1988, nutritionists have understood that this usually negative aspect of sugar becomes a real quality when it is necessary to accelerate the muscle re-construction of glycogen, mainly used up during a soccer match. If a player ingests at least 60 grams of table sugar dissolved in water as soon as the match ends, within the first two hours he can re-construct up to nearly 7 millimoles of glycogen per hour per every kilogram of muscle tissue, that is more or less 7% of all the glycogen present in full stores. It is important to underline that, if sucrose is ingested some hours after the match - and not immediately after the end of the competition - it would take a longer time for glycogen to re-construct. The same thing happens if a player ingests the same amount of fructose, instead of sucrose or glucose.

If a player ingests another 60 grams of sugar two hours later, he can be sure that 25 to 30% of muscle glycogen will have been re-constructed in his muscles only four hours after the end of the match. Moreover, if he has a diet rich in carbohydrates at the main meals following the competition, as shown in the box on page 28, his muscle glycogen stores will be full for the match he is going to play two or three days later. On the contrary, if the player has a mixed diet, neither 48 nor 72 hours can be enough to re-plenish muscle glycogen completely, especially if some of the meals taken mainly consist of proteins, (different kinds of meals, fish, cheese...).

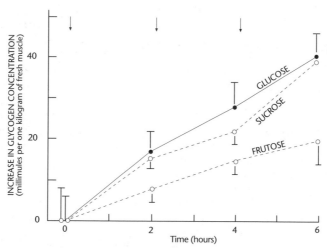

Muscle glycogen re-construction after ingesting approximately ten grams of glucose, sucrose or fructose both immediately after the match and two hours later. Glucose helps muscles to re-construct up to 7 millimoles of glycogen per every kilogram of muscle tissue per hour; similar re-construction rates can be obtained with sucrose; while these levels are considerably lower when players ingest fructose. Modified by Blom and his colleagues, 1992.

Branched-chain amino acids

In the last few years, nutritionists have realized that athletes can recover much more rapidly from physical efforts if they ingest branched-chain amino acids, substances representing nearly 20% of the proteins we usually ingest with nutriments. Since they are 'essential amino acids', our diet should provide a suitable portion of these substances every day, so as to avoid possible disorders and diseases. The three essential amino acids consisting of a carbon branched chain (valine, leucine and isoleucine), play an important role, if ingested in sufficient quantities, 9 grams at least. They help to avoid sudden drops in anabolic hormones concentration in the blood, (see the paragraph on page 78 and the box on page 80-81) and to rapidly repair the lesions occurring in muscle fibers during the efforts of the match.

2

DIET AND TRAINING

While referring to the relationship between diet and training, it is immediately necessary to underline that players are confronted with many different situations, according to their category, but also according to the different periods of the year and of the soccer season. During pre-season training sessions, for instance, most players train twice a day, and training loads are often higher than those they will have during the rest of the season; moreover, they are often obliged to practice in particular weather conditions, characterized by high environmental temperatures. All these factors inevitably influence the way players choose their foods and drinks. In the course of a normal championship season, only professional players usually practice twice a day - as well as some young players playing on major division clubs, but only when they have no school commitments.

Moreover, because of their school timetable, it is often difficult for most young players to have a traditional midday meal, especially in winter, when training sessions generally take place earlier in the afternoon. On the other hand, most players cannot have a normal evening dinner - in terms of contents and/or time - because they usually practice late in the afternoon or at night.

THE DIET IN THE PRE-SEASON PERIOD

In the pre-season period, that is starting from late July for professional players and from mid August for most other players, players are usually subjected to hard work: professional players generally practice twice or even three times a day, while amateur players usually have one single training session which is often more strenuous than regular sessions during the season.

This fact determines the need for players to have a suitable intake of calories and nutrients in the right proportions, which is not a real problem in general, as well as the need not to overload their digestive system during training periods. Furthermore, players should choose diets helping them to digest easily and to be in the best physical condition and completely efficient during training sessions. Even though many players can often digest perfectly, even when they eat foods that would generally cause various problems to many other people because of their own characteristics or because they are combined with other nutriments, it is important to consider that our digestive system is not always absolutely efficient. And it would really be a pity to give up or to postpone a training session just because of diet errors!

Rehydration is another nutritional factor which is particularly important in the pre-season period, characterized by the highest temperature levels of the year. Even though many teams train in cool places, players inevitably lose a great quantity of liquids while perspiring during everyday training sessions. For this reason, it is necessary for them to re-plenish water and salts they lost during their practice. Moreover, they should check their rehydration, at least by keeping their body weight under control (see the box on page 28).

Breakfast

If the training session takes place in the morning - especially early in the morning, to avoid the hottest hours of the day - players cannot have a traditional breakfast. When there is a particularly demanding practice, especially when using highly lactic acid exercises, players should eat breakfast at least one hour before the beginning of the training session and their first meal should exclude fats. It is necessary to avoid butter and croissants and other fatty breakfast cakes since they are always less digestible than bread. Players should also exclude coffee with cream, as it takes a long time to digest and it can cause gastric acidity. Those players suffering from gastritis or other disorders concerning the digestive system, should avoid drinking coffee altogether. It takes a long time to digest milk too, and, for this reason, every single player should consider whether to drink it or not, according to his own past experiences. Moreover, some people find it difficult to digest citrus fruit juices. Among the most common beverages people generally drink at breakfast, tea is the one which usually causes the least problems.

A good breakfast should include substances providing

carbohydrates, above all in the form of starch; on the contrary, simple sugars should be ingested in small amounts. Only fructose can be assimilated in larger quantities with no particular problems appearing, but in some cases, it can cause diarrhea if its intake exceeds 50 grams; so, it is better to eat bread with a little marmalade or a little honey. The ideal breakfast - easy to digest for a morning training session - should consist of bread with marmalade and tea, ingested in moderate portions. The longer the period between the end of one's breakfast and the beginning of one's practice, the more it can be like the meal described in the paragraph on page 37 and the more generous the portions.

Many players will feel that they were cheated out of something, when they are asked to eat little at breakfast; but, if necessary, they can 'recover their loss' by eating fruit at the end of the morning practice.

One last consideration. I think it useful for athletes practicing aerobic sports - for Marathon racing in particular, Arcelli, 1989, - to get accustomed to training in the morning without having breakfast, so as to stimulate fat consumption. The same thing cannot be suggested to soccer players whose muscles draw most of the energy they use during training from carbohydrates. Those who often suffer from digestive disorders even if they eat little, ingesting foods which generally create no particular problems, should have breakfast earlier in the morning, even though many players prefer getting up at the last minute, and should also reduce their food and drink intake drastically, or eat just half or one of the dietetic bars especially produced for athletes. However, I think that when digestive disorders persist, the player can face his training session without having breakfast. If necessary, he can eat some dietetic tablets rich in carbohydrates if his physical efficiency while practicing is seriously impaired because of a possible drop in glycemia levels.

The midday meal

I believe it is advisable for soccer players to start their midday meal with a dish of mixed vegetables, either cooked or fresh, dressed with vinegar, or lemon, and little extra virgin olive oil. Vegetables are one of the best gifts nature offers us; and it would be a real shame not to use them regularly! If players spend their pre-season training period all together in a dormitory, while entering the dining room they

REHYDRATION CONTROL

How can players check that they have re-plenished the water they lost while training?

The simplest way is to keep one's body weight under control regularly, in standard conditions. It should be checked every morning, a few minutes before having breakfast and wearing only one's underpants. The scale should always be the same and should ensure an accurate weighing system; moreover it must be placed on a level surface.

Soccer players have always been asked to check their body weight every day during the pre-season period; and in the past, when people still believed that losing weight always meant slimming down, the more players' weight decreased, the more athletes and coaches were satisfied.

Today, on the contrary, everybody knows that a sudden drop in one's body weight is never a positive factor and must be considered suspiciously. Actually, even if athletes practice strenuous exercise and eat little, they can use up only a small amount of fats, ten grams of fat a day at most; for this reason, this sudden decrease in the body weight is likely to have a precise meaning: the player in question is dehydrated, that is he has not re-plenished part of the lost water. It is advisable for a coach to question the athlete about his condition: if he has had physical disorders such as consti-pation or diarrhea, if he has eaten too much, if he has intentionally drunk less than usual. Unfortunately, there are still some persons who believe it is useful, if he feels particularly tired out or experiences unusual sensations and so on.

It is important to measure the body fat percentage - by means of plyo-metrics for instance, see chapter 3, - not only at the beginning and at the end of the pre-season period, but also every time a particular player sud-denly loses weight.

Moreover, it is fundamental to consider that sometimes players are like-ly to keep water in their muscles at the beginning of the pre-season train-ing period and, therefore, their body weight can increase by a few ounces; the muscles of these athletes are usually 'tough' and sometimes ache when you massage or touch them - as the trainer can attest.

A dehydrated player is not in the best condition to practice well; in particular, if he lacks more than one kilogram of body water, his autono-my is considerably reduced, his efficiency is prematurely undermined dur-ing training and he is more vulnerable to various accidents.

In any case, it is advisable for those players suffering from a consider-able decrease in their body weight to undergo further medical investiga-tion.

should immediately find various bowls on the table, containing different kinds of vegetables: cooked or raw carrots, tomatoes, cucumbers, boiled potatoes, spinach, zucchini and so on.

In this way, players avoid stuffing themselves with bread and water - that is what usually happens for particularly hungry people, who are anxiously waiting for their meal - and eat foods providing vitamins, salts, oligoelements, fibers and a lot of water. And everybody knows how important it is in this period to help the re-plenishing of the large amount of water lost while perspiring.

I remember the first time I suggested that players begin their meals with a generous portion of vegetables many years ago. I had some difficulties in persuading them, but the players and the coaching staff soon understood that it was the right habit.

Theoretically, after eating vegetables, players should have the so-called one course meal, with a basis of carbohydrates (pasta or rice) when there is a training session in the afternoon - or rich in proteins (all kinds of meat, sliced ham, cheese) if they are not going to practice in the afternoon. But I think this should be reasonable above all for overweight players (see page 32) or for those suffering from digestive disorders, since athletes practicing strenuously, will hardly accept giving up a complete meal, carbohydrates + proteins.

Moreover, I am persuaded that players should also be allowed to have a dessert: a piece of cake, without cream or custard, or a fruit ice cream. However, it is important that both the first and the second course of the meal provide the lowest quantity of fried or cooked fats possible. When the players have already eaten fruit at the end of their training sessions, they do not need to eat it at the end of their main meals, since it is sometimes likely to cause various problems when it is ingested after other nutriments; but, in my opinion, this cannot be considered as an absolute prohibition.

This is the ideal midday meal suggested in the pre-season training period:
- fresh or cooked vegetables, dressed with vinegar, or lemon, and extra virgin olive oil;
- a portion of pasta or rice, with extra virgin olive oil, or butter, or fresh tomato sauce;
- a portion of lean meat, chicken or turkey, or a portion of fish cooked with no fats, or the lowest quantity possible; or sliced ham or cheese;

- an ice cream, a fruit ice cream is preferable, or a piece of apple pie or cake without cream or custard;
- mineral or carbonated water and bread.

During and after training

During training - even in the shortest pauses of the session - players should always have drinking water available, or, still better, specific beverages for athletes; among these drinks, players should prefer those having low sugar and salt concentrations, that is those which stimulate a more rapid rehydration (for further explanation, see Chapter three).

At the end of the training session, players should be offered fresh fruit. Actually fruit, as well as vegetables, is one of the best gifts nature gives us; it helps us to re-plenish lost water, and it also provides fibers and extremely useful nutrients.

Players should be allowed, or even urged, to have some mineral or carbonated water bottles in their bedrooms, to drink in the afternoon, before training, or at night, after the evening dinner. I cannot emphasize enough the importance of suitable rehydration for soccer players.

The evening dinner

The evening dinner should allow players to completely replace all the substances lost in the course of the day. As to overweight players exclusively, their dinner should consist of vegetables and one single course. As a rule, the other players can follow the suggestions given for the midday meal, that is: a generous portion of mixed vegetables preceding the first and the main course, containing the minimum amount of fried or long cooked fats, and then a dessert. However, I believe that players can be allowed to choose among different kinds of sauces for pasta or rice and among different varieties of main courses. In any case, if they want to make some exceptions to the rule, or better: one single exception at a time, in other words, if they want to eat something different from their usual diet they should prefer a meal distant from the training session: the midday meal if they do not practice in the afternoon; the evening dinner in other situations, particularly if there is no training session the next morning.

THE 9 RULES FOR THE PRE-SEASON DIET

1. The pre-season period usually coincides with the hottest months of the year and training sessions cause players to perspire profusely every day.

2. Players should have the possibility of drinking during the breaks - even if very short.

3. It is necessary for players to stimulate their re-hydration at the end of the training session; for this purpose, it is important to eat fresh fruit and drink sports drinks.

4. It is better to begin every main meal with a generous portion of fresh and/or cooked vegetables.

5. Players should constantly check their re-hydration, checking their body weight regularly - every morning at least.

6. It is fundamental to consider that, during the pre-season training period, many teams usually practice twice, or even three times, a day and, therefore, the intervals between one session and the following one are extremely short. For this reason, it is important to put athletes in the condition to train without suffering from digestive disorders.

7. When there is very strenuous training in the morning, players cannot eat too much at breakfast and they should ingest easily digestible foods. Therefore, white coffee and toast should be avoided; it is advisable to exclude butter, too.

8. At the main meals, at midday in particular, players should choose those foods which are easy to digest; for this reason, it is better to exclude foods with fried or long cooked fats, cold cuts, fatty meat, sauces and so on.

9. Those players who have a high body fat concentration cannot slim down too quickly; furthermore, restrictions to their calorie intake cannot be excessive in a period when training loads are usually the highest in the year.

Overweight players -
Players having excessive body fat

Most players begin the pre-season training period in good physical condition. As a matter of fact, many of them keep on practicing by themselves during their vacation and they are particularly attentive to their diet. As a consequence, there are less and less players putting on weight during their long vacation. Moreover, many athletes keep the same body weight they had at the end of the previous season, even though plyometrics sometimes shows that their muscle mass has decreased by two or three pounds and the fatty mass has increased by as much.

Usually, a slight increase in one's body fat does not require any dietetic measure, since it often tends to disappear in a few weeks. Only in case of excessive fat is it advisable for those players to reduce their calorie intake: obviously, they cannot exaggerate, otherwise they would risk their possibility to practice in their best condition.

Besides reducing table sugar and sweets intake to minimum levels, it is important to suggest that both the midday and the evening dinner should consist of one single course (one-course meal) following a generous portion of vegetables, still better if dressed with little oil. These two meals should obviously be complementary, that is: if the first meal had a basis of carbohydrates, the second one should be rich in proteins and vice-versa. On the contrary, there is absolutely no need to reduce the water intake.

Dietary supplements during
the pre-season training period

Besides the drinks especially produced for athletes, are there any other dietary supplements players should systematically ingest during the pre-season phase?

The fifth chapter will deal with the features and the real importance of all the different supplements in detail. Here, we just want to touch upon this subject. I would like to underline that - because of hard training during the pre-season period - it is often necessary for players to ingest:

- **vitamin C:** players can choose to ingest one gram at one single time as soon as they get up in the morning, or very small doses at different moments during the day. Some dietitians recommend polyvitamin-polymineral supplements. The smaller the portion of fruit and vegetables players eat every day, the larger the quantity of supplements they should ingest. The same principle is valid for vitamin C as well;

- **branched-chain amino acids:** they play an important role, controlling the possible excessive increase in catabolic hormones and the relevant considerable drop in anabolic hormones due to strenuous exercise (see Chapter 4).
- **creatine:** training overloads cause our body to lose a lot of creatine. For this reason, those players who have low muscle creatine concentration should take this substance orally, so that they help their body to bear more strenuous physical exercise (see the paragraph on page 79).

Always referring to the most suitable nutriments included in the table on page 22, the above-mentioned meals should follow the following pattern:

- pasta or rice, either in broth or not, with raw oil or raw butter or fresh tomato and vegetables;
- different kinds of fresh or cooked vegetables, preferably boiled potatoes and/or boiled carrots with little oil,
- vegetables can be eaten before or after the main course; one main course of any kind, providing it is a moderate portion and it contains little fat;
- one dessert, but without cream or custard;
- bread as much as you like; water as much as you like; one coffee for those who are accustomed to it.

Even though I insist upon the importance of a high carbohydrate diet throughout the week, this does not mean that I consider proteins to be of little importance for soccer players. Foods having a high protein content (various kinds of meat; fish and shellfish; milk, cheese and yogurt; eggs) play a crucial role in the nutrition of human beings in general and of athletes in particular; as will be explained in the paragraph on page 63-66, devoted to vegetarians. Those who usually eat few of these nutriments run the risk of

THE 10 RULES FOR A SUITABLE DIET DURING THE SOCCER SEASON

1. During the soccer season the diet of soccer players should respect those rules helping them to reach and then preserve a general well-being.
2. Moreover, some meals should have the special purpose of increasing glycogen stores in muscles; these meals must provide a large amount of carbohydrates and, on the contrary, a moderate quantity of proteins and very few fats. Pasta, rice, bread, potatoes, desserts are the most suitable nutriments for these meals.
3. The meal immediately after the competition and, if necessary, the meals on the next day should be rich in carbohydrates, so that players can be sufficiently efficient from the physical point of view during the first training sessions of the week.
4. Moreover, the main meals (two at least, or still better four) the breakfasts and the snacks players have on the days preceding the match should consist of foods rich in carbohydrates.
5. If the match is always played on the same day of the week, players should observe a precise week cycle, considering not only the match and the training sessions, but also their diet, consisting of some meals particularly rich in carbohydrates - Immediately before and after the competition - and others in which the carbohydrate intake is not strictly necessary.
6. This week cycle should also include some meals which must be particularly easy to digest, especially for those players suffering from digestive disorders, for instance: the meals before training sessions.
7. The main meals consisting mostly of carbohydrates are usually the easiest to digest; a one-course meal, consisting of one main course, pasta or rice, even in a much more generous portion than usual, is often particularly digestible, provided that - obviously - it does not include a lot of fats.
8. When the player is going to practice in the morning, his breakfast must be very easy to digest; he should avoid white coffee in particular.
9. The habit of ingesting vitamin C, and other antioxidant vitamins such as polyvitamins and polyminerals, is an excellent precaution for athletes; as a rule, these substances are particularly useful if the player does not eat a lot of vegetables and fruit regularly.
10. Many dietitians believe that, among all the different dietary supplements - in addition to the supplements mainly consisting of vitamins and/or minerals, and to the beverages especially designed for athletes, those with a basis of branched-chain amino acids and creatine play a very important role during the soccer season.

suffering from various deficiencies.

Therefore, it is advisable for players to have normal portions of foods high in proteins at the main meals distant from the competition, not immediately before or after the match.

The meals preceding the training session

As a rule, the table we suggested for a meal rich in carbohydrates is useful also for the meal preceding a training session or a competition, when it takes place in the afternoon (see the paragraph **'Immediately before the match'** on page 11).

Actually, the foods high in carbohydrates are usually easier to digest than those rich in protein, and much easier than fatty nutriments.

The meal preceding every training session should obviously consist of moderate amounts of foods, in relation to the interval between the end of the meal and the beginning of practice. In general, it is more difficult for players to have a sufficiently long interval of time if they have to practice twice a day. However, those players suffering from digestive disorders can resort to the common 'one-course meal', consisting of nourishments high in carbohydrate, pasta or rice, thus reserving a generous amount of proteins for the evening dinner, unless this is the period when players should pay particular attention to their glycogen stores.

With regard to morning training sessions, it is important for players to eat easily digestible foods at breakfast. According to my own experience, I would like to underline that when a player vomits, or suffers from digestive disorders, in the course of the morning training session, this is very often due to the fact that he probably drank white coffee and a slice of toast at breakfast.

As to particular cases - for instance, young players who often have no time to eat a complete midday meal - see the paragraph **'The nutrition of young soccer players'** on page 36. Furthermore, the section **'Practical problems of players'** on page 40 is particularly interesting for players who usually practice late in the afternoon or at night, and, therefore, cannot have their evening meal at the usual time.

Supplements during the soccer season

According to our modern knowledge, only on particular occasions during the soccer season should soccer players regularly ingest dietary supplements other than:

- drinks for athletes, already prepared or which can be prepared with special powders;
- those consisting of vitamins and minerals, alone or combined together;
- protein supplements, for instance: creatine, branched-chain amino acids and, if necessary, carnosine and glutamine.

Some paragraphs in Chapter 4 will deal with these dietary supplements in detail and with other supplements advisable exclusively for particular players in particular situations (see Chapter 3).

THE NUTRITION OF YOUNG SOCCER PLAYERS

As you can observe in the table below, young athletes' daily needs for some particular nutrients (proteins, calcium, iron, vitamin C) - per every kilogram of one's body weight - are higher than adults' needs.

Recommended daily levels for the intake of some particular nutrients - in 12 to 18-year-old soccer players and in adults - per every kilogram of body weight.					
Age	12	14	16	18	Adults
proteins g/kg/a day	1.47	1.63	1.31	1.21	1.07
calcium mg/kg/a day	32	23.5	18.5	16	12.5
iron mg/kg/a day	0.3	0.25	0.2	0.15	0.15
vitamin C mg/kg/a day	1.2	0.9	0.7	0.65	0.65

However, according to my own experience, one of the most common dietary problems among young soccer players, their mothers and their coaches, is the midday meal when the training session takes place in the early afternoon. Usually, young players do not practice in the morning; this can occur in some particular clubs especially in the summer period and, sometimes, during Christmas holidays.

The digestive disorders of those who have not digested or have eaten nothing for a long time

While professional players have the possibility to manage their own spare time in part, at least, and therefore can nearly always choose the time for their meals, young players often have great difficulties and the midday meal is generally a problem for them. Furthermore, it takes a very long time for some young players to move from one place to the other and for this reason, they are often obliged to miss their midday meal or, at best, to eat one or two sandwiches.

Therefore, some young players are likely to suffer from gastric disorders, something lying heavy on their stomach, nausea, vomit, or from more general problems, dizzyness or loss of strength, due to the fact they have not digested yet. Other players, on the contrary, feel particularly weak because - after experiencing digestive disorders during one of the previous training sessions - they have eaten nothing for a long time, maybe since the night before.

I believe that, in these cases, it is fundamental not only to care about the midday meal, but also to reconsider the dietary habits of the whole day.

Breakfast and the mid-morning snack

First of all, young players should learn to have a rather abundant breakfast, even if this causes them to get up 10 to 15 minutes earlier than usual. There is still a large number of young people who eat absolutely nothing at breakfast and this is a great mistake. It is undoubtedly very useful for them to get used to ingesting a certain amount of complex carbohydrates, in the form of bread, with a thin layer of marmalade or honey; it would be still better for them to eat whole meal cereals, in flakes or other forms. They should be accompanied by a drink: tea, milk or coffee with cream. Yogurt, too, is particularly recommended.

It would be very useful to start breakfast drinking a glass of citrus fruit juice: in winter it is possible to prepare it at any time, squeezing fresh oranges, while in other periods you can use canned juice with no sugar added.

During the mid-morning break at school, young players should have a snack: they should avoid prepared common snacks, very rich in low quality fats and sugar, and prefer fresh fruit.

A suitable diet for the midday meal

When he has eaten a rich breakfast early in the morning followed by a mid-morning snack, the young player can eat less than usual at lunchtime. He could have a portion of pasta or rice exclusively.

But it often happens that young players cannot go back home or are obliged to give up their midday meal completely, either because the interval between the end of the meal and the beginning of the training session is too short, or because it takes such a long time for them to get from one place to the other, as was explained earlier. In this case, they can eat a cheese or sliced chicken sandwich immediately after their school lessons, along with one or two fruits, or a dietetic bar for athletes; for this reason, their mid-morning snack should be more abundant: for instance, it can consist of one or two sandwiches.

However, they can even miss their midday meal completely if the morning breakfast and the snack together have already provided the adequate number of calories. Young athletes do not run the risk of losing their strength while they are practicing. It is really absurd and unjustified to believe that energy stores can deplete totally during the training session. Because of this wrong belief, many young soccer players do not give up their meal although they haven't enough time to digest it; as a consequence, they are undoubtedly more vulnerable to digestive and other general disorders, connected to the fact of practicing physical activity while the digestion is still underway. They will have time to balance the amount of substances ingested and substances lost immediately after the training session and at the evening dinner!

The diet for young players having very little time

In short, considering what we said before, young players who are

THE 10 RULES FOR THE NUTRITION OF YOUNG SOCCER PLAYERS

1. Young players' daily needs for proteins, calcium and some vitamins - per every kilogram of one's body weight - are higher than adults' needs.
2. The most commonly felt dietary problem among young players is undoubtedly the great difficulty in having a normal midday meal when there is an afternoon training session.
3. In the winter season in particular, when days are naturally shorter, the interval of time between the end of the school lessons and the beginning of the training session is very restricted; during this interval, young athletes are also obliged to move from school to their house and from home to the training ground, and these transfers often take a long time.
4. If there is little time between the end of the meal and the beginning of exercise, players are more likely to suffer from digestive disorders while they are practicing.
5. The shorter this interval, the greater the attention they should give to their dietary choices.
6. In case of at least a two hour interval, players have the possibility to have a normal meal; anyway they should eat less than usual: for instance, a portion of pasta or rice with raw extra virgin olive oil, or raw butter or fresh tomato.
7. If they have less time, less than two hours, and it really takes a long time for them to move from one place to the other, they should be more attentive to their nutrition in the previous hours: this means that they should have a rich breakfast and eat a mid-morning snack.
8. If they have no time to go home after school, they can eat one or two sandwiches with fresh cheese and sliced chicken or turkey while they are moving from school to the training field.
9. If the interval of time is still shorter, young athletes should take care to eat something more for the mid-morning snack and not to eat anything before the training session, or just one dietary bar for athletes, with a very low fat content.
10. However, young athletes, and their parents, must understand that it is not necessary to have a real complete meal to have a good physical performance during practice.

going to practice in the afternoon immediately after their school lessons can choose among three possible diets:

First possibility, when they have at least a two hours' interval between the end of the lessons and the beginning of the training session and it does not take a very long time for them to move from school to their house and from home to the training field:

- **breakfast:** citrus fruit juice; whole meal cereals and/or bread, with marmalade or honey; tea or milk or white coffee and/or one yogurt;
- **mid-morning snack:** fresh fruit, an apple and an orange for instance;
- **midday meal:** pasta, or rice, with raw extra virgin olive oil or butter, or fresh tomato.

Second possibility, when they have a two hours' interval between the end of their school lessons and the beginning of the training session, but they have some problems concerning their transfers from one place to the other:

- **breakfast:** abundant, like the example above;
- **mid-morning snack:** fresh fruit;
- **midday meal:** one or two sandwiches with sliced chicken or turkey, or fresh cheese.

Third possibility, when the interval between the end of school lessons and the beginning of practice is still shorter:

- **breakfast:** abundant, like the example above;
- **mid-morning snack:** one sandwich with sliced chicken or turkey and one cheese sandwich;
- **midday meal:** one dietary bar for athletes, with a very low fat content and little sucrose, or nothing at all. In this case, young players can keep some dietary bars - mainly consisting of carbohydrates - at their disposal, in case their physical efficiency is impaired during exercise because of a drop in glycemia levels.

PRACTICAL PROBLEMS OF YOUTH AND COLLEGE PLAYERS

Which are the main differences between the nutrition of youth and college players and professional players?

From various points of view, one could not imagine so many differences. It is true that, unlike what many people believe, there is

40

not one single diet effective for, and recommended to, all athletes; actually, since the effort the human body has to endure is different from one situation to the other, also nutritional needs inevitably vary. However, considering the general features of the kind of effort the body has to perform, it is also true that players practicing soccer for their own pleasure exclusively are not substantially different from professional players.

The differences between professional and youth and college players

Therefore, there cannot be any substantial differences between a professional player's diet and a youth and college player's nutrition - in terms of qualitative choices of foods and nutrients, at least.

However, there can be some differences from other points of view; but I do not want to give the impression that professional soccer players need a higher calorie intake, since they practice more than others. Actually, there are possibly some amateurs whose jobs necessitate a considerable expenditure of energy for eight hours or more on work days. In these particular conditions, therefore, the problem should be tackled individually with every single athlete.

There is another quite common problem: the production of excessive amounts of free radicals, also connected to strenuous physical activity (see the specific paragraph on page 61). These atoms, or groups of atoms, represent one of the causes for the increasing risk of those kinds of injuries known as 'repetitive micro-trauma injuries' and 'overload injuries', affecting above all soft tissues or elements, tendons, ligaments and bursae. Therefore, those who usually practice more strenuously, or work harder, should pay much more attention to their nutritional choices, in particular to a suitable daily intake of antioxidants, starting with vitamins - important substances inhibiting the oxidation reaction by removing oxygen free radicals. Meanwhile, it is useful to avoid, or reduce to minimum levels, those foods generally enhancing the production of free radicals.

When players practice at night

It is fundamental to consider that most soccer players - excluding professional athletes, some young players and a few others - practice at night, when most people are usually having dinner. This fact

41

often causes problems to these athletes. Eating before the training session is not really advisable, since it is difficult to practice physical activity when food has just reached the stomach; actually, physical effort can stop their digestion, especially in winter, when the temperature is very low in some particular regions, and induce nausea, vomiting and even much more general disorders. On the other hand, many soccer players fear that practicing without having eaten for a long time is counterproductive as well, since this could cause a sense of weakness.

Well, how should they behave in this case?

First of all, soccer players should realize that having eaten nothing, or nearly nothing, for a long time - since the midday meal, for instance - does not necessarily impair their body's efficiency. Then, they should think about reconsidering the nourishments distribution throughout the day.

From this point of view, breakfast plays a crucial role. Actually, very often soccer players do not have the possibility of eating at home at midday; therefore, instead of a really complete meal, they are obliged to eat just a sandwich. All the more reason to have an abundant breakfast, and not to merely drink a cup of coffee as many people usually do. Breakfast should include something to drink, milk, if they can digest it; tea or coffee, and a suitable amount of carbohydrates such as bread with a thin layer of marmalade or honey and whole meal cereals (see the paragraph on page 51).

Then, it would be better to have a mid-morning snack consisting of fruit or one yogurt. A midday complete meal consisting of first course, main course, side dish and fruit is advisable only for those who do not suffer from digestive disorders and/or for those who can eat just a cold dish after the evening training session. Moreover, it is evident that they should avoid foods which take a long time to digest or are difficult to digest, starting from those rich in fried or long cooked fats, and they should pay attention to suitable nutriments combinations.

In the middle of the afternoon, they should take a snack, preferring fresh fruit to yogurt, for instance. If somebody really feels the need for something more nourishing, a sandwich with chicken or turkey, or fresh cheese is suggested. Where players have at least a two hour interval before the beginning of the training session, this undoubtedly enables them to accomplish their digestion and, on the other hand, it is an important factor for those who still believe that having eaten nothing for a long time necessarily impairs their body's efficiency during exercise: once more, I would like to repeat that this is a groundless fear!

If players cannot have any kind of snack in the afternoon, they can eat a dietary bar for athletes - highly digestible and with a very low fat content - shortly before starting practicing. If they have eaten nothing at all for a long time, they should keep some carbohydrate bars at their disposal in case their physical efficiency is impaired because of a drop in glycemia levels.

Before speaking about what players could eat after their evening training session, it is first of all necessary to imagine a common situation. Most families are not willing to prepare dinner once again some hours after the other members have eaten, for a player who usually practices after work and often comes back late at night, probably because the training field is very far from home. Those who have a microwave oven can warm up previously cooked foods; the others can only eat a cold dish such as cheese, cold cuts, eggs or canned food.

If players make the right choices, these nourishments can be included in their diet, provided that they are ingested only twice or three times a week and combined in many different ways.
Moreover, it fundamental to avoid excessive amounts of animal fat. Therefore, players should limit their cheese and meat intake. There are no limits as to the water intake, apart from those imposed by one's own common sense.

I would like to remind you that the evening dinner should include any kind of vegetables - better fresh vegetables; in other words, soccer players should at least learn to dress their dish of vegetables, if they are not going to learn how to cook their own meals!

THE IDEAL BODY WEIGHT

Sometimes, athletes practicing different sports disciplines need to lose body fat simply to be allowed to compete. Suffice to think of those athletes practicing particular sports, such as, weightlifting, the light category in rowing, boxing, judo and other combat sports, in which there are weight limits they cannot exceed. Also in other sports disciplines, in particular: middle-distance and long distance racing, including the marathon, an excess of body weight negative-

THE 10 RULES FOR THE NUTRITION OF YOUTH AND COLLEGE PLAYERS

1. From a qualitative point of view, there are no substantial differences between professional players' nutritional needs and youth and college players' requirements.
2. As far as the calorie intake is concerned, there cannot be any important differences between professional players' needs and youth players' requirements. Actually, professional players usually practice more than the others, and, therefore, they spend more time on the playing field, but among youth and college players' there are some whose job implies a considerable expense of energy and calories eight hours a day.
3. Many soccer players train at night, after 6 p.m., or even after 8 p.m.
4. Therefore, these players cannot have dinner at the usual time, when the others generally do.
5. Furthermore, they can not eat before the training session because they may suffer from gastric or more general disorders during exercise.
6. Not only should these players put off their evening meal to a later time, after the training session, but they should reconsider their nutrition throughout the whole day.
7. First of all, it is advisable for them to have an abundant breakfast.
8. Moreover, they should take a mid-morning snack and have a complete midday meal.
9. Then, two hours before the training session, they can have a snack, consisting of fruit or even a sandwich and something low in fat; if players cannot have their afternoon snack, they can however eat one dietary bar for athletes shortly before training.
10. It is not necessary to have a hot dish after the training session; a suitable combination of cold foods can help players to complete their daily nutritional requirements.

ly affects the performance, since the energy expense increases as the body weight grows.

It is not so important to care about fractions of a pounds in soccer; however, some pounds of body fat in excess undoubtedly impair one's abilities during the game. This is due to various reasons: practically, it is like wearing a weighted belt round one's waist or carrying a rucksack on one's shoulders during exercise. This burden causes players to sprint and jump less than usual and affects their ability to accelerate and to move sideways; moreover, physical efforts being equal, athletes get tired more rapidly; it is like wearing a pair of insulating coveralls, since the fat layer lying under the skin makes it more difficult for the body to expel the heat produced by muscles; therefore, thermo-regulation, that is keeping the body temperature within acceptable limits, becomes much more difficult.

For all these reasons, it is necessary to check that players have no excess fat, if they do it is worthwhile judging the importance of a suitable slimming diet - obviously, a diet especially designed for athletes.

WHAT IS ONE'S IDEAL BODY WEIGHT?
In the past, dietitians in soccer circles were used to speaking of top-condition body weight; they referred to the player's body weight coinciding with a period of top physical condition and they used it as a reference to understand if it was necessary for him either to increase, which happened very seldom, or decrease his body weight at a particular time.

In reality, apart from the body weight, it is much more reasonable to measure the fat mass concentration; actually, in this way it is possible to get much more useful information. Top physical efficiency is not a direct consequence of one's top-condition body weight or of one's fat mass concentration; it is influenced by different factors, among which genetics, suitable nutrition and previous exercise are the most important ones. Then, training and nutrition inevitably affect one's body weight and fat mass concentration.

Slimming down and losing weight
In soccer, there are still some persons muddling up these two different concepts: slimming down and losing weight. As a consequence of a soccer match players can lose several pounds, but this

does not mean they have slimmed down by several pounds. As a matter of fact, slimming down means something particular: losing fat. The pounds players usually lose after any physical effort mainly consists of water - leaving their body in the form of perspiration and of glycogen, in low concentrations, that is the animal starch occurring in muscle and liver cells, and from which muscles draw the energy they need to work during a competition. As it will be explained later, players only lose just a few ounces of fat doing such exercise!

This fact should help us understand how illogical is the choice is of those who go jogging - maybe in August, in the hottest hours of the day - wearing heavy or even rainproof clothes, deceptively believing this is the best way to lose excess fat.

3

THE SOCCER PLAYERS' DIET

The first chapter mainly dealt with players' nutrition before, during and after the competition, while in the second chapter the attention is totally focused on the connections between nutrition and training practice. In these two important moments, the match and the training session, it is advisable for players to observe some specific dietary rules and criteria. Otherwise, their physical performance is very likely to be impaired during exercise. However, apart from these particular cases, athletes' nutrition should always be healthy and well-balanced, since it definitely helps them to reach a condition of full physical and psychological well-being, which is important for everyone of us and especially for athletes. Moreover, adequate nutrition of the body makes players less vulnerable to general disorders, sickness and injuries which can often be prevented by respecting some rational dietary suggestions.

There are some people who believe that it is necessary to eat a variety of foods in order to feel good but I think that this kind of statement can lead to bad mistakes. If on one hand it is completely wrong to restrict the choice to very few foods and always prefer the same ones, as shortage of some particular nutrients is very likely to appear in these cases, on the other hand it is not proven that constant variations in one's diet are really beneficial - also because there is such an incredible variety of foods today we could ingest the same kinds of nutrients while also eating nourishments of different shapes and tastes.

In short: it is very important to diversify one's diet, but it should be done by observing specific reasonable criteria.

The main errors to avoid

After studying the dietary habits of people living in industrialized countries, a number of national organizations and international agencies have finally come to the conclusion that we should

introduce some important changes in our diet, in order to enjoy general well-being and good health. In particular, we should:
- reduce fat intake
- reduce table sugar intake
- ingest more fibers

There are undoubtedly many athletes who already respect these rules - who do not ingest too many fatty substances, control their sugar intake and eat foods high in fiber - but there are still many players who do not; therefore, these basic suggestions are especially for those who still make considerable dietary errors.

Reducing fat intake

The first paragraph in the appendix of the book clearly shows that there are different kinds of fats. In particular, it is fundamental to reduce the ingestion of animal fats - like butter, cream, sausages, fatty meat, beef, pork, mutton, poultry, - as well as the consumption of cheese, whole meal and dairy products in general. Fats derived from animals living on land are richest in saturated fatty acids, raising the production of cholesterol-LDL. LDL or low-density lipoproteins are responsible for arterial diseases, restriction and loss of elasticity, and increase the danger of cardiac problems and other circulatory disorders.

Oils (extra-virgin olive oil is far better than the other varieties) should be used to flavor foods, provided it is in moderate quantities and, if possible, uncooked; it is advisable to alternate red and pork meat with white meat like chicken and turkey; moreover, don't forget to trim fat off meat and use very little cooking fat. Some dietary research suggests we should eat fish and other fish products three times a week, since they help to maintain blood fluid and have many other beneficial effects. Breaded, fried or long cooked fatty foods should be excluded completely from one's diet or consumed very seldomly.

Reducing sugar intake

Reducing sugar intake means reducing the amount of sucrose in particular, that is common table sugar which should be considered as a chemical substance more than a real nutriment. Unlike all the other nourishments, it contains neither vitamins nor minerals and therefore is said to provide 'bare calories'. The ingestion of foods and

THE 10 DIETARY ERRORS TO AVOID

1. Today, most people tend to take in too much fat, too much sucrose or table sugar, and to reduce, on the contrary, the amount of foods rich in fibers, like vegetables, fruit, legumes and whole meal cereals.

2. As far as fats are concerned, players should limit animal fats in particular; it is therefore advisable to reduce the consumption of butter, cream, sausages, fatty meat, as well as cheese, whole milk and other dairy products.

3. Only very rarely should athletes eat fried foods or nutriments containing long cooked fatty substances.

4. It is important to limit condiments; extra-virgin olive oil must be preferred to any other kind of oil.

5. It is recommended to choose very lean beef and pork; red meat should be regularly alternated with chicken and turkey. Moreover, it is important to avoid cooking fats and to accurately trim fat off meat.

6. The diet should include fish or other fish products three times a week.

7. Players should limit their alcohol intake.

8. Players should reduce their sucrose (table sugar) intake and therefore limit, or completely avoid, sweet and carbonated drinks, as well as desserts, candies and so on. In particular, they should never ingest more than a few grams of sucrose at a time.

9. It is fundamental to eat more foods high in fibers, like vegetables, fruit, legumes and whole cereals. In addition to fibers, many of these nutriments also provide other important substances helping general well-being, like minerals, vitamins and various antioxidants.

10. Breakfast should provide foods with a high fiber content, like whole meal cereals; moreover, the main meals should always include a portion of vegetables, while it is advisable to eat fresh fruit at the mid-morning and mid-afternoon breaks. The diet should include five portions of foods rich in fibers every day.

drinks high in sugar in the course of the whole day should be limited. Furthermore, it is advisable not to take in more than ten grams at a time, since such a quantity would suffice to raise glucose and insulin concentrations in the blood. From this point of view it is far better to use fructose, the sugar occurring in some varieties of fruit and having the same taste as sucrose.

It is important to remember that players should not reduce their sugar intake in the post-match period if another match is going to be played within a few days; as was explained in the first chapter - they need to drink as much as two cans of a drink containing sucrose or glucose immediately after the first match.

The importance of fibers in the diet

Dietary fibers, or roughage, are not attacked by digestive enzymes and, therefore, are not digested, so that they are passed on to the large intestine, where they add to the bulk of the feces to be voided. This gives the intestinal muscles something to grip, increasing their efficiency and preventing the need to strain; moreover, they help to maintain glucose and cholesterol blood concentrations within healthy levels. Epidemiological research shows that those who regularly ingest a suitable amount of foods with a high fiber content are less vulnerable to various diseases (see chart on next page). This is the reason why it is worthwhile taking whole meal cereals and muesli at breakfast, vegetables and/or legumes at the main meals and fresh fruit at the mid-morning and mid-afternoon breaks. An important British researcher suggests ingesting five portions of foods rich in fibers to be chosen among vegetables, fruit and legumes every day, since they also provide, though in different concentrations, very beneficial substances to our health, like minerals, vitamins and various antioxidants.

THE RATIONAL DISTRIBUTION OF FOODS DURING THE WHOLE DAY

Irrational distribution of foods in the course of the whole day is a very widespread error. For instance, it is important to eat a hearty breakfast, while it is advisable to limit one's food intake at midday. Moreover, training sessions and competitions necessarily influence nutrition, as was clearly explained in the first and second chapters. On all other occasions, players should follow what is recommended in the following paragraphs.

FRUIT AND VEGETABLES
THE FIVE-PORTION RULE

It is common knowledge that vegetables, fruit and legumes are very beneficial to our health and help the body to be less vulnerable to various diseases, while little precise information is usually given on the suitable amount to take in. English professor Carol Williams has gradually worked out a rule which allows us to understand whether we have ingested the optimum amount of these foods on a particular day or not: according to her rule, we should take in five portions of 80 grams each day. Moreover, professor Williams has also drawn up a table which helps us to easily calculate what a portion of one particular nutriment corresponds to.

Nutriment	A portion corresponds to:
Big fruits (pineapple, watermelon, melon)	one wedge
Medium-sized fruits (orange, banana, apple, pear)	one fruit
Small fruits (apricot, plum)	two fruits
Berries (strawberries, raspberries, blackberries)	one cup
Stewed fruit (e.g.: apples or canned fruit, e.g.: peaches)	three spoonfuls
Dried fruit (raisins)	twelve teaspoons
Citrus fruit juice or fruit juice	one glass
Greens (broccoli, spinach)	two spoonfuls
Roots (carrots, turnips)	two spoonfuls
Stewed legumes (chick-peas, beans, lentils	two spoonfuls
Small vegetables (pease or corn kernels)	three spoonfuls
Salad (lettuce, endive, tomatoes)	one dish

Breakfast

If players are not going to practice in the morning, they had better eat a hearty breakfast, provided that any excess of fat and sucrose is avoided. The ideal breakfast should therefore consist of:

- a glass of citrus fruit juice, or one citrus fruit, to prepare the stomach to receive the other nutriments; citrus fruits provide very important nutrients like vitamin C, various antioxidants and salt;
- a nourishment with a high carbohydrate content, like bread or toast with a little honey or marmalade; it is advisable to avoid butter and danish pastries in particular. Whole meal cereals are

very important because of their high fiber and mineral content but should not necessarily replace bread;

- something to drink like tea, coffee and/or milk; milk can be replaced by a cup of yogurt;
- if necessary, a nourishment mainly providing proteins, - one boiled egg, one slice of ham or light cheese, for instance. Athletes must avoid eating these kinds of food when they need to digest in a short time or when they suffer from digestive disorders.
- Eating different varieties of fruit (fresh fruit is recommended) is the best solution, when players feel the need or the desire to diversify their breakfast.

EATING, DRINKING, SLEEPING

Everybody knows that some particular drinks and foods ingested during the evening meal, or in the hours immediately after the meal, are likely to either stimulate or disturb sleeping at night, while very few persons really know how or why the evening food intake can influence rest. For instance, there are some particular substances, mainly occurring in some drinks, which directly act on the nervous system. The most common example is undoubtedly coffee: it contains caffeine, as well as all the other xanthines, starting from theine in tea, which has well-known stimulating effects and often disturbs quiet sleeping. On the contrary, there are some other beverages like chamomile-tea or other herb tea, lime, tangerine, lettuce tea..., which contain well-known substances having a completely opposite effect to caffeine and other xanthines, since they help one to sleep.

Stimulant or soothing natural substances can also be found in some particular foods. As the saying goes 'cheese is gold in the morning, silver in the afternoon and lead at night'; in reality, different cheeses contain considerable amounts of tyramine, sleep's 'enemy'. Some nourishments with a high protein content, on the contrary, are very rich in tryptophan, an important amino acid stimulating sleeping; this is the reason why some believe that eating meat at the evening meal helps to sleep better.

The diet definitely interferes with normal sleep, since sleeping disorders also result from digestive disturbances. While we are sleeping, the organs and the systems in our body (the muscles, the heart, the circulation...), usually work at a lower rhythm or do not work at all. When a person eats too much and/or takes in foods which take a very long time to be digested, his digestive apparatus has to work very hard, thus interfering with normal sleep. Therefore, those who want to have a good sleep should exclude gravies, fried foods, particularly elaborate courses, nourishments containing long cooked fats... from their evening meal.

Moreover, there are some foods which usually cause sleeping disorders to a very restricted number of people, while, in general, they are absolutely harmless; therefore, it is fundamental for everyone of us to carefully identify the nutriments which should be excluded from the diet because of their negative effects.

Why are there such a number of different personal reactions?

There are numerous reasons for this. First of all, as far as digestion is concerned, there are considerable differences from one person to another; but there are many other elements to take into consideration. Coffee, for instance, is supposed to stimulate sleeping in some persons; according to one of the main hypotheses, this seems to be possible because these persons discharge their last energies in the period of maximum excitement occurring between drinking coffee and falling asleep.

Anyway, it is important to remember that the psychological aspect is the key to understanding one's own disposition to getting to sleep quickly. As a matter of fact, there are many people who are persuaded they cannot peacefully go to sleep if they drink a cup of coffee late in the afternoon; but, some researches have definitely proven that these persons can not fall asleep when they drink a cup of decaffeinated coffee, which they believe is normal coffee, while they are very likely to immediately get to sleep after drinking a glass of milk or a cup of lime-tea added with a huge dose of caffeine of which they are unaware.

Therefore, those who suffer from sleeping disorders, as far as soccer players are concerned, the night before the match in particular, should always follow their own usual habits and rituals: reading, watching TV, as well as drinking a cup of herb tea, or a cup of coffee for those who really feel the need.

THE 10 RULES FOR A RATIONAL DISTRIBUTION OF FOODS DURING THE WHOLE DAY

1. Not only is it important to control the diet from both the qualitative and the quantitative point of view, but it is also fundamental to distribute the nutriments in a very rational way throughout the whole day.

2. Most people, both sedentary people and athletes, tend to miss breakfast or eat very little in the morning; this is a very bad mistake, unless there is a training session immediately afterward.

3. Breakfast should consist of: nutriments with a high carbohydrate content, bread, for instance, with a little marmalade or honey; something to drink, like tea, coffee or milk (which can be replaced by yogurt); a glass of citrus fruit juice or, in winter, one citrus fruit, which should be ingested immediately at the beginning of the meal. Whole meal cereals or muesli are highly recommended.

4. The midday meal should be very easy to digest, especially if players are going to practice early in the afternoon.

5. It is advisable not to overload the digestive apparatus if we want to be perfectly efficient while we are studying or working.

6. The midday meal can be a one-course meal, consisting of one main course, preferably pasta or rice, - a more generous portion than usual is allowed - preceded or followed by a dish of cooked or fresh vegetables.

7. If there is no need to lose weight, the evening meal can include: one pasta course, one main course, a portion of vegetables and one dessert.

8. The evening meal can also be a one-course meal. It is advisable to alternate carbohydrate and protein intake; therefore, if the midday meal mainly provided carbohydrates (pasta or rice) the evening meal should consist of food with a high protein content (a dish of red or white meat or a fish course).

9. Coffee or white coffee and a croissant, or any other snack, usually containing unhealthy fatty substances, should be avoided at the mid-morning break; it is far better to prefer fresh fruit.

10. The mid-afternoon break should consist of fresh fruit or a cup of yogurt.

The midday meal

The midday meal should not be too difficult and long to digest, especially for those who are going to study, work hard or practice in the afternoon, and for all those who need to maintain top physical and psychological efficiency in the hours immediately after the meal.

From this point of view, it is first of all necessary to reduce fat content as much as possible, and avoid fried and long cooked fats in particular (read the box on page 49). Some athletes should not eat any fruit at the end of the meal, since it prolongs the time for digestion. Moreover, players should try to avoid wrong combinations of foods, which means they should not ingest nutriments requiring different kinds of digestion in the same meal, see the paragraph concerning food combinations on page 56. When they need to digest more rapidly or when they usually suffer from digestive disorders in the afternoon - unpleasant disturbances which considerably impair the performance while studying or working - they can resort to the so-called one-course meal. It consists of either one first course (pasta or rice), or one main course (meat, fish, mixed cheeses, or eggs) - a more generous portion than usual is allowed - followed, or still better preceded, by a dish of cooked or fresh vegetables. As was clearly explained in the second chapter, the midday one-course meal should provide a high carbohydrate content if players are going to practice in the afternoon.

The evening meal

The evening meal is supposed to fill the gap between the calories spent throughout the day and the calories taken in while eating breakfast, the midday meal and any possible snack. If the player has had a hearty breakfast in the morning and a one-course meal at midday, and he is not overweight, he should eat a meal including:

- one pasta or rice course or soup;
- one main course: meat, fish, eggs or cheese;
- one side-dish: cooked or raw vegetables;
- the dessert: a piece of angel food cake or some fruit ice-cream.

The snacks

The mid-morning or the mid-afternoon snacks should consist of fresh fruits. As previously pointed out, fruit tends to prolong the time necessary for digestion when it is ingested at the end of a meal, but also at the beginning or in the course of the meal. Therefore, it should be avoided, especially if the athlete is going to practice or usually suffers from digestive disorders. However, fruit is particularly beneficial to our health and should be ingested regularly and abundantly; for this reason, it is highly recommended for the mid-morning and mid-afternoon snacks. A cup of yogurt is another possible healthy solution.

FOOD COMBINATIONS

There are some players who easily digest everything they eat, including commonly heavy foods. However, things are sometimes very likely to change as time goes by: in the last few years, I have directly noted that, in many athletes, the digestive system sometimes 'ages' more quickly than muscles or the heart. As a matter of fact, some athletes, who usually enjoy excellent physical condition, are very likely to develop digestive disorders by the age of 24; therefore, they begin by carefully selecting the foods they can eat before physical exercise and by excluding those which - according to their past experience - could impair their health again. Only later on can they realize that any wrong food combination is very likely to prolong the time for digestive processes.

However, combining some particular nutriments can sometimes have beneficial effects, since the biological value of what is ingested can be enhanced considerably.

Food combinations negatively affecting the digestive process

Digestive fluid's ideal features - that is the elements which help more rapid and whole digestive processes - are quite different from one group of foods to another. However, by simplifying the reality, it is possible to point out some typical situations.

If a person eats some starchy nutriments - a dish of pasta, for instance - a reduced amount of acid gastric juices is secreted within the first two hours; in this way, ptyalin, the enzyme present in the saliva and responsible for the initial stages of starch digestion - so that it immediately mixes with pasta during mastication, can work effectively. But, if the person ate some meat, or another food with a high protein content, immediately after the pasta course, the stomach lining membrane would secrete large quantities of strong acid gastric fluid; in this way, ptyalin would be immediately inactivated in the stomach, thus slowing down starch digestion.

In a very similar way, digestive processes can be further delayed by the combination of different varieties of nutriments high in protein - like milk and meat, milk and eggs, or meat and eggs, and so on. As a matter of fact, every single food requires different digestive conditions, concerning, for instance, the time needed to produce more acid gastric juice.

Therefore, for the digestion to be more effective and rapid, it is fundamental to avoid combining protein (meat, cheese, and eggs) and sugar (candies, cookies, and bread with honey or marmalade) since sugar inhibits the secretion of those gastric juices providing the enzymes necessary for protein digestion.

Fruit delays the digestion of most foods, but it especially inhibits the secretion of pepsin, an enzyme that catalyses the breakdown of proteins to polypeptides in the stomach. If on one hand fruit is very beneficial to soccer players since it provides vitamins, mineral salts, fibers and other important substances, on the other hand it is better to avoid eating fruit at the end of the meal preceding physical exercise, whether a training session or a match. It is much more advisable to eat fruit far from the main meals, for instance at the mid-morning or mid-afternoon snacks, or before going to bed. A hearty breakfast including fruit exclusively would be a healthy solution.

The one-course meal

I was the first person in Italy to suggest to athletes the so-called one-course meal some years ago, that is a meal consisting of one first course, or one main course preceded or followed by a portion of mixed vegetables. Since that time, though, I have realized that some athletes cannot adopt this solution. I immediately want to point out that I have not changed my mind: I merely want to suggest that this may not be the best solution for everybody. Actually, I firmly believe that the one-course meal should be recommended in most cases, especially when the athlete needs to digest very quickly. This is very important for those who need to be perfectly efficient early in the afternoon, because they are going to study, work or practice physical exercise. For instance, the young soccer player, (see the paragraph '**The nutrition of young soccer players**' in Chapter two) who comes home from school at about 2.30 p.m. and often begins practicing at 3 or 3.30 p.m. - especially in winter, when days are very short and the training session must end before it gets dark. In this case, the one-course meal should consist of a portion of pasta or rice and the player should avoid even the vegetable course for those who usually suffer from digestive disorders. It is much easier to digest one single food than different varieties of nutriments, since each one has its own peculiar digestive features for those who need to slim down or tend to put on weight. It is proven that a one-course meal, even though the portions are more generous than usual, provides a considerably lower amount of calories than a whole meal, including the first course, the main course and the side-dish.

The combinations which enhance the biological value of nutriments

Many firmly believe that animal proteins are irreplaceable, they are actually known as first-class proteins. Vegetable nutriments contain incomplete proteins, which means they lack one or more essential amino acids, 9 important substances which cannot be synthesized by the liver and must be provided ready-made in the proteins of the diet.

Lysine, for instance, is an essential amino acid which cannot be found in bran pasta which, contrary to what many people think, has a considerable protein content (more than 10% in some cases) nor in all the other nutriments deriving from cereals, that is from wheat, as well as from rice, corn, oats.

Though legumes, beans, peas, chickpeas, lentils, and broad beans, have a high protein content, which can even account for 18 to 24% of their dried weight, they are very poor in methionine, one of the nine essential amino acids.

Fortunately, cereals are particularly rich in methionine and legumes in lysine; therefore, if cereals and legumes are combined together, in the same course or in the same meal, the body is provided with a suitable protein supply, whose biological value is considerably enhanced.

It is interesting to note that some decades ago people were preparing foods which met these important requirements without being aware of the detailed content of nutriments or of the real needs of the body, basing their diet only on direct observation of what was happening around them. Pasta and beans, or broad beans, or lentils, and rice with peas are just two examples of their long tradition. Therefore, combining cereals and legumes is one of the possible solutions to provide the body with the suitable amount of proteins, and it is especially recommended either for those who need to reduce their animal protein intake or for vegetarians.

Milk and cereals or polenta and cheese are two other examples of food combinations which considerably enhance the quality of the protein content of every single nutriment.

Vitamin and mineral absorption

The vitamins and minerals occurring in foods are often absorbed only in part. The percentage of absorbed substances directly depends on what is being digested in the intestine at that moment. The most popular example is iron; as will be explained in the paragraph **'Iron and the athlete's anemia'** in the next chapter, many soccer players are more vulnerable to developing anemia because the balance between the amount of iron absorbed and that of the lost iron is upset. There are some particular nutriments which, combined with foods with a high iron content (meat, for instance) can disturb the absorption of iron by the intestine. They include: milk, eggs, bread, coffee and some vegetables. Other nutriments, especially vitamin C, can help iron be absorbed in the body.

Furthermore, there are some other food combinations which can either prevent or help vitamins and minerals pass from inside the intestine into the bloodstream. Alcohol, for instance, is an obstacle to the absorption of both vitamin A and its precursors, provitamins; on the other hand, both vitamin A and its precursors enhance the absorption of zinc, an oligoelement occurring in fish, which is particularly important for athletes. Vitamin D, also occurring in fish, promotes the absorption of calcium from the intestine, while spinach contains some specific substances which prevent calcium from being absorbed. Some other greens - like cabbage, cauliflower, broccoli - provide particular substances which make iodine absorption much more difficult.

THE 10 RULES FOR COMBINING FOODS

1. Each food requires a particular kind of digestion; for instance, gastric juices having specific features.

2. Digestion is more likely to be slow and difficult when two kinds of foods requiring different digestive processes are ingested in the same meal.

3. It takes a much longer time for the stomach to digest a meal combining starch (pasta) and protein (meat).

4. Digestion can be further prolonged when two different foods with a high protein content are combined together: milk and meat, for instance, or milk and eggs, or meat and eggs.

5. In the same way, combining protein (meat, cheese or eggs) and sugar (candies, cookies, bread with honey or marmalade) can have negative effects on digestive processes.

6. Eating some fruit at the end of the meal often prolongs the digestion period.

7. Therefore, it is much easier to digest a one-course meal, obviously consisting of easy digestible foods, than a whole meal including the first course, the main course and the dessert. Actually, the one-course meal (it is advisable to prefer the pasta or rice course - with little condiment - and a portion of cooked or raw vegetables) is a helpful solution for those who need to digest quickly and for players who are going to practice a very short time later.

8. The one-course meal is particularly recommended to those who usually suffer from digestive disorders and to those who need to lose weight.

9. Combining cereals and legumes, like pasta and beans or rice and peas, for instance, considerably enhances the biological value of the protein content of each nutriment; this is the reason why these protein combinations can effectively replace animal proteins (meat, for instance).

10. The combination of two different foods often causes one particular vitamin or one particular mineral, occurring in one of the two nutriments, to be absorbed more or less effectively; the absorption of the iron occurring in meat, for example, is considerably enhanced by vitamin C and usually hindered by milk, eggs, bread or coffee.

FREE RADICALS: HOW TO FIGHT THEM OFF

Free radicals are extremely reactive molecules because of their unpaired electrons, incessantly produced in the body during normal metabolic processes. These molecules are the cause, or one of the main causes, of several disorders, including serious diseases. Moreover, they are one of the main factors in ligament, tendon and muscular injuries, which are by far the most common injuries' in soccer - 'repetitive microtrauma injuries' and 'overload injuries' in particular.

The negative effects of free radicals are mainly fought by antioxidants, important substances that slow the rate of oxidation reactions. Some of them are produced in the body (endogenous antioxidants) while others are generally assimilated in the diet (exogenous antioxidants).

Free radicals: their main effects

Oxygen is of vital importance for the human being to survive; but, paradoxically, it can become an enemy of the human body and of some specific structures in particular. Free radicals, very reactive substances which are particularly harmful to our health, can originate from oxygen. Consequently, free radicals are produced in much greater amounts in those who practice physical exercise and therefore consume more oxygen. Other factors can stimulate the production of these molecules; they include: air pollution, smoking, ionizing radiation (including sun radiation), some drugs, some particular fats in foods, alcohol and so on.

Free radicals are said to be the cause, or one of the main causes, of a number of disorders and illnesses, including the most serious diseases like cancer and some forms of atherosclerosis, characterized by the evident narrowing and thickening of arteries, thus increasing the probability of developing heart disease and other circulatory disorders. Moreover, they enhance the aging of the tissues, of the organs and of the whole body, and affect various structures - like cell membranes and mitochondria membranes - as well as molecules of critical importance in the nucleus such as DNA, proteins and so on. Some researchers are persuaded that free radicals also play a crucial role, combined with other local and general factors, in inducing some tendon, ligament and muscular injuries. Obviously, the reference is made neither to 'direct trauma accidents' - which are very common in soccer and which are mainly due to the violent impact between one part of the body of the athlete who suffers the trauma and an external object, the body of another athlete in most cases - nor to 'indirect trauma injuries', like ankle or knee sprain from excessive rotation or flexion of the joint beyond maximum limits.

These molecules are supposed to be involved also in muscular lesions - usually known as sprains and contractures in the language of coaches and athletes - and in what is commonly defined as late muscular pain, which does not affect muscles while practicing or immediately after, but only 24 to 48 hours after physical exercise. This is very common during the pre-season training period. Furthermore, free radicals often induce 'repetitive microtrauma injuries' and 'overload injuries', which are the result of continuous repetitive stresses acting on a part of the body: these mechanical stresses would be absolutely harmless by themselves, but, since they combine their effects together, they often result in real lesions.

Antioxidants

Our body fortunately produces particular substances which allow us to defend ourselves against free radicals; these molecules endogenous antioxidants - are specific enzymes, like glutathione peroxidase and peroxide-dismutase. There are better known as scavengers, since they literally 'sweep away' free radicals, or, better, they defeat or reduce their negative effects.

When a small amount of free radicals generate in the body, these endogenous antioxidants - which are usually produced in larger quantities in those who regularly practice physical exercise - are generally able to defeat their aggressive attack. But if free radicals proliferate in the body endogenous antioxidants may not be enough to defend the body.

Therefore, it is fundamental to introduce other free radical 'enemies', that is exogenous antioxidants which are mainly provided by foods. They include very powerful substances occurring - even though in very different percentages - in many varieties of fruit and vegetables. Vitamins are by far the commonest exogenous antioxidants: in particular vitamin C, vitamin E and beta-carotene, which is also called provitamin A since it changes into vitamin A in the body.

In order to prevent a number of diseases - cancer or atherosclerosis, for instance, which are very often ignored by athletes, even by 'the oldest' ones, since they still feel young - and to reduce the risk of developing tendon, ligament or muscular injuries, soccer players, especially the oldest ones, since they have gradually overloaded their locomotor apparatus and are therefore more vulnerable to injuries, should regularly eat fruit and vegetables, preferably fresh, and live a healthy life, trying to avoid smoking, drinking and exposure to air pollution.

Vegetable nutriments provide the body with vitamin exogenous antioxidants. Many varieties of fruit and greens are particularly rich in these substances (see the table on page 64).

The oligoelements occurring in exogenous antioxidant molecules and which must be introduced from outside include: selenium, in the glutathione peroxidase molecule; manganese, entering the superoxide dismutase molecule in the mitochondrion; and copper and zinc, entering the superoxide dismutase molecule in cytoplasm. Other non-vitamin exogenous antioxidants, which have been given considerable importance in the last few years are found in tomatoes, summer lemon, extra-virgin olive oil, red wine, green tea (very common in Japan), garlic, cabbage and so on.

For those who are not used to eating fruit and vegetables at all or eat very little amounts of them, (read the box on page 52), it is undoubtedly important to regularly take in vitamin C, either in tablets or in powder to dissolve in water, as well as polyvitamin and polymineral substances providing very useful oligoelements like selenium, manganese, copper and zinc. Shortage of these oligoelements would make the synthesis of endogenous antioxidants diffiult.

VEGETARIAN PLAYERS

In the last few years, I have met an increasingly high number of athletes who have suddenly decided to become vegetarians at a certain moment of their lives. Nine out of ten of them, at least, say they have made this choice for their health, ('Meat is bad for my health'), and only a small minority present ethical reasons, ('I cannot accept that animals are killed to satisfy our needs exclusively'). However, in most cases I usually come into contact with them for one main reason: they have become anemic.

As a matter of fact, those who do not eat meat and, meanwhile, do not take care of ingesting foods with a high iron content run the

FRUITS AND VEGETABLES RICHEST IN VITAMIN C, VITAMIN B AND VITAMIN A OR IN BETA-CAROTENE

VITAMIN C
(in milligrams per 100 grams of edible substance)

Fresh Fruit		Vegetables and greens	
kiwi	90-150 mg	parsley	140-170 mg
citrus fruits	40-50 mg	peppers	120-200 mg
strawberries	40-55 mg	broccoli	50-100 mg
raspberries	25 mg	spinach & cauliflower	50-60 mg
melon	20-35 mg	cabbage	40-80 mg
persimmons	20-25 mg	lettuce	50-60 mg
bilberries	20 mg	endive & celery	30-35 mg
pineapple and bananas	15-20 mg	tomatoes & leeks	20-25 mg
apricots	15 mg	asparagus & chicory	15-20 mg
cherries	12 mg	radishes	15 mg

VITAMIN A
(in mirograms of vitamin A or in equivalent amounts of carotene per 100 grams of edible substance)

Fresh Fruit		Vegetables and greens	
apricots	350-500 mg	carrots	1200 mg
persimmons	200-250 mg	parsley	1000 mg
yellow melon	200 mg	yellow pumpkin	600-800 mg
yellow peaches	100 mg	spinach	500-600 mg
oranges	70-75	chicory & lettuce	220-260 mg
bananas	40-50	celery & broccoli	200 mg
watermelon	30-40	green cabbage & endive	200 mg
plums	20-30	peppers	100-150 mg
tangerines & clementines	25 mg	tomatoes	50-150 mg
bilberries & cherries	20-25 mg	asparagus	80 mg

VITAMIN E
(in mirograms of alpha-tocopheral per 100 grams of edible substance)

Fresh or oily fruits		Vegetables and greens	
hazel-nuts and peanuts	1000-3000	broccoli & peas	150-200 mg
blackberries & raspberries	350-500	tomatoes and leeks	100 mg
apples & pears	200-400	spinach & lettuce	50 mg

risk of iron deficiency and, therefore, of developing the so-called 'athlete's anemia'.

Is meat really bad for our health?

We are often told that athletes should not eat red meat, but is it really bad for their health? Should we really feel at fault every time we eat a steak?

It is immediately necessary to specify that there are no rational reasons for forbidding red meat to healthy people. However, it is fundamental to advise people against eating excessive amounts of some particular kinds of meat for one specific reason: the varieties which are apparently leanest inevitably contain a certain percentage of fat. Those who usually take in much animal fat are more likely to experience an increase in cholesterol and other fat concentrations in the blood, LDL - low-density lipoproteins - concentration in particular, so that they are much more vulnerable to developing arterial disorders and, consequently, heart diseases, including infarction, and circulatory disturbances. However, from this point of view, there are many possible reactions to animal fat intake which can be very different from one person to another. Furthermore, I also want to underline that meat provides 15 to 20% of proteins and, as a consequence, eating too much meat could require considerable overwork to remove excess proteins, which would possibly result in physical disorders in some cases.

Red meat can therefore be included in the diet, but it is advisable to avoid eating it twice a day and every day, that is 14 times a week, especially when the diet already provides other foods with a high protein content (cream, butter, cold cuts, whole milk and plain yogurt, cakes with custard). When we eat a lot of meat, we should take the necessary precautions: first of all, it is fundamental to choose the leanest varieties of meat and reduce cooking fats, or avoid them completely, as well as trim fat off the meat before eating it. Moreover, red meat should sometimes be replaced by white meat like chicken and turkey, especially when cholesterol and LDL blood concentrations are particularly high; it is also advisable to eat fish twice or three times a week, at least. In conclusion: in order to guarantee perfect health in future, one does not need to become vegetarian.

The diet of vegetarian players

Is it possible to be vegetarian and practice a top-level sport discipline like soccer?

It is undoubtedly possible in many cases, like in those disciplines involving prolonged physical performance. Manuela Di Cent, for instance - cross-country skiing Olympic champion - is almost completely vegetarian, and Bettina Sabatini, who finished in fifth place at the New York Marathon, is 100% vegetarian.

I would like to point out something of critical importance: becoming vegetarian does not merely mean excluding meat from one's diet without changing all the rest. In this way, deficiencies in some important nutrients - iron and proteins, in particular - are very likely to appear, thus increasing the risk of general disorders and even serious diseases. Moreover, the body is gradually deprived of creatine, a substance occurring in meat exclusively; this deficiency does not cause any particular disorder or disease but it considerably impairs one's physical efficiency.

Remember that athletes' daily needs for protein, iron and creatine are much higher than sedentary people's requirements, even if there are considerable differences from one sport discipline to another; this is the reason why entirely vegetarian athletes must learn how to eat properly.

Proteins can be absorbed both through animal nutriments different from meat, eggs, milk, cheese and other dairy products, and through vegetable foods combined with cereals (see the paragraph on page 58).

Every meal should also provide a suitable amount of iron; vegetable nourishments contain a kind of iron which can be absorbed in lower percentages than animal iron, further details will be given in the next chapter. It is advisable to eat whole meal cereals at breakfast, preferably combined with citrus fruit juice, which considerably enhances iron absorption. Moreover, the main meals should always include generous portions of vegetables, especially the varieties richest in iron like spinach and other greens; almonds, oily fruit, yolk, cocoa and brewer's yeast also have a high iron content.

Furthermore, it is advisable to sometimes avoid drinking beverages which disturb iron absorption, such as coffee, tea, milk and red wine; while orange juice, or any other citrus fruit juice, is highly recommended.

Shortage of creatine is a serious problem mainly concerning vegetarian athletes practicing explosive-force disciplines, like sprinting and hurdles in track and field, and other sport disciplines - such as soccer, tennis and other team games - where periods of heavy physical exercise alternate with periods of little effort or no physical work at all. Creatine is a nitrogenous compound that occurs in muscles and whose concentration cannot exceed 4.6 grams per every kilogram of muscle (for further details read the paragraph and the box concerning creatine in the next chapter). Small amounts of creatine are also produced in the body every day, with differences from one person to another; unfortunately, these amounts are usually much lower than the percentages athletes inevitably lose while practicing. This is the reason why muscle creatine stores do not deplete when the diet regularly provides the body with suitable amounts of this important substance. Unfortunately for vegetarians, meat (beef and pork, poultry and all the other varieties, as well as fish - excluding shellfish) is the sole nutriment providing creatine and no other food can have this particular property.

In conclusion, vegetarian athletes constantly have lower muscle creatine concentrations than usual, up to 30% lower than maximum levels; therefore, it is almost impossible for them to practice some sport disciplines, including soccer, at top levels in terms of physical performance if they do not have a well-balanced diet. In particular, that diet should regularly include foods with a high protein and iron content, as well as the only nutriment providing creatine, that is meat; creatine supplements, combined with carnosine, if necessary, are a unique alternative solution.

THE 10 RULES FOR VEGETARIAN ATHLETES

1. Those who have decided to completely exclude meat from their diet should be aware that their body is more likely to be short of some important nutrients, iron and protein deficiencies in particular.

2. Most meals should provide proteins with a high biological value and therefore include foods having these special properties like cheese and eggs.

3. Milk or yogurt is recommended at breakfast. If the athlete usually eats a lot of cheese, he had better use skim milk, and skim yogurt, instead of whole milk. For the same reason, it is also advisable to choose foods with a low fat content.

4. Legumes provide considerable amounts of iron and protein; the diet should therefore include peas, beans, lentils, chickpeas and soy beans.

5. Apart from legumes, there are some other vegetable nutriments providing iron even though in a form, non-heme, which cannot be absorbed in the same way as meat ferroheme. For this reason, it is important to eat such foods as parsley, spinach and other greens, whole meal cereals, almonds and all the different varieties of oily fruit several times a week. Yolk, brewer's yeast and cocoa also have a good iron content.

6. There are some particular drinks which considerably disturb the absorption of iron occurring in nutriments; they include coffee, tea, red wine and milk. Therefore, it is better to avoid combining these beverages with foods having a high iron content.

7. It is advisable to drink water at the main meals; if the athlete does not suffer from digestive disorders, he can even drink citrus fruit juices whose vitamin C content considerably helps iron absorption.

8. Legumes' proteins perfectly combine with cereals', so that their total biological value is considerably enhanced; this is the reason why the same meal or the same course should include both legumes and cereals like pasta, bread, rice and corn.

9. Fruit and vegetables provide many important nutrients, like vitamins and oligoelements, and therefore daily fruit and vegetable intake is particularly beneficial to our health: each main meal

should include a generous portion of vegetables, while it is better to eat fruit at the mid-morning and mid-afternoon snacks, and drink citrus fruit juice, combined with whole meal cereals, at breakfast.

10. Vegetarian athletes have lower muscle creatine concentrations; since creatine is an important reserve of energy for muscle contraction, creatine deficiency is a serious problem because there is little ready-made 'fuel' to use, it is more difficult to re-plenish oxygen deficit and muscles are much more vulnerable to the negative effects of lactic acid. For physical performance to be really effective, the vegetarian athlete needs to take in creatine supplements, preferably combined with carnosine, another important substance which only occurs in meat.

4

SUPPLEMENTING THE DIET

Dietitians usually talk about supplementing athletes' nutrition, or about dietary aid programs, when referring to nutriments, drinks and other special substances athletes are suggested to take in some particular conditions or situations, and which are not included in a common diet.

In reality, athletes do not always need to introduce these extra substances; however, supplements are sometimes the easiest or the most effective way either to solve or to prevent a problem.

WHY IS IT IMPORTANT TO SUPPLEMENT ONE'S DIET?

Many athletes regularly ingest dietary supplements, like vitamins, minerals, amino acids or some particular carbohydrate and peptide supplements. But is it really necessary for them to absorb these substances?

The effects of strenuous and frequent physical exercise (enhances consumption; stimulates losses of salt and water while sweating; increases muscular turn over and oxidation reactions) can undoubtedly stimulate the body's need for some particular substances usually occurring in foods. Moreover, absorption of some of these substances in the intestine can be further reduced as a consequence of physical effort. Therefore, the body is more likely to experience severe deficiencies which immediately impair physical performance and may result in real disorders or diseases. For instance, shortage of glutamine weakens the body's immunity to infection, while iron deficiency is the main cause of anemia.

When a well-balanced diet is not enough

Isn't it enough for athletes to accurately choose the most suitable food combinations either to prevent or cure these deficiencies?

In some cases, in reality, dietary supplements cannot further help the athletes who already have an adequate nutrition or the diet

THE MAIN FACTORS FOR WHICH
ATHLETES NEED TO SUPPLEMENT THEIR DIET
(by E.G. Di Monteventano, 1994, modified)

There are many reasons for which an athlete really benefits by supplementing his diet with vitamin, mineral, special carbohydrate, amino acid, peptide... supplements:

• while practicing strenuous and frequent physical exercise, it is more difficult for the body to absorb some nutriments and the need for some particular substances can grow considerably; deficiency of some important elements immediately impairs the physical performance and often results in pathological conditions.

• theoretically, all the substances necessary for the body could be introduced with the diet; but it is fundamental to underline that foods sometimes provide a minimum quantity and this would mean:

- eating large amounts of these particular nutriments, for instance, several ounces or even some kilograms of meat to introduce a suitable amount of creatine or branched-chain amino acids,
- ingesting many other substances which are useless or even harmful to the body - especially if they exceed certain doses, saturated fats, for instance, when a person eats too much meat to take in creatine or branched-chain amino acids,

• food processing techniques, like preserving or cooking processes, reduce the real content, and therefore the real properties, of some substances, like some vitamins, for example.

• some ingredients occurring in one particular nutriment are absorbed in very low percentages in the intestine, like iron non-heme, occurring in vegetable foods.

• in order to properly choose the most suitable foods so as to provide the body with the substances it really needs, the athlete should have a wide knowledge of the main aspects of dietology.

could completely satisfy the needs, provided the athlete is really familiar with dietology, dietary rules and food contents so as to perfectly identify the most suitable nutriments and the perfect quantity he needs. As was explained in the previous chapters, players should not trust selective hunger, that is the mechanism by which one would sometimes ingest the right foods providing the substances he really needs. This process can sometimes have misleading effects: it often happens that some persons, whose body balance between sodium and potassium is already upset because of severe sweating, eat great amounts of fruit to re-plenish part of the lost water, thus further aggravating the situation.

Moreover, it is important to remember that the substances which should be absorbed either to prevent or cure dietary deficiencies cannot be provided by one single food in abundant quantities. They are always combined with other molecules which could be useless or even harmful to the body, and which often need a very long digestive process to be removed.

Suffice to think about branched-chain amino acids. For instance: most varieties of meat contain nearly 4% of them. Consequently, if a person added some extra 200 grams of meat to his diet in order to increase branched-chain amino acid intake, he would provide the body with little more than 2 grams of valine, the same amount of isoleucine and 3 grams of leucine, that is a much lower total quantity of branched-chain amino acids than athletes' daily requirements. Meanwhile, he would also introduce nearly 30 grams of other amino acids - which are very likely to be useless for the body, which needs to metabolize these substances and remove the nitrogenous molecules they produce from the kidneys - and a considerable amount of unhealthy saturated fats, often causing serious disorders.

The real content of some particular substances

There are some practical problems concerning the real content of some particular substances. As a matter of fact, cultivation techniques as well as preserving and cooking processes usually impoverish the real content of some nutriments, so that the real value is sometimes lower than it appears in common dietary tables. Moreover, other substances generally have a very low bio-availability: only 2 or 3% of iron non-heme - occurring in vegetable foods -

THE 8 REASONS FOR
SUPPLEMENTING ONE'S DIET

1. Dietary supplements are sometimes the easiest and/or more effective way to either cure or prevent some disorders.

2. Frequent, strenuous and/or prolonged physical exercise sometimes stimulates the need for some specific nutrients.

3. Frequent, strenuous and/or prolonged physical exercise raises the consumption of various substances, enhances the loss of water and salt, stimulates muscular turn over, increases the number of oxidation processes and so on.

4. Frequent and strenuous and/or prolonged training sometimes reduces the ability of the intestine to completely absorb some important nutrients.

5. Theoretically, the diet itself could provide all the nutrients which are often introduced with dietary supplements.

6. Some substances that the athlete needs in some particular situations are much easier to absorb if they are introduced with supplements.

7. If a player wants to take in one specific nutrient through the diet - without using dietary supplements - he is sometimes obliged to eat large amounts of one particular food, for example, various portions of meat to increase creatine or branched-chain amino acid intake. In this way, he also ingests large quantities of other substances which are useless for the body and even harmful to his health.

8. For the diet to provide all the nutrients the body really needs, the athlete must have a wide knowledge of every aspect of dietology.

Nutrition for Soccer Players

Supplement	Purpose (real or apparent)
Re-hydrating drinks	• preventing dehydration and unbalance or electrolytes
Products providing carbohy-drates (powder, tablets, beverages) or other substances to feed energy stores, short or medium-chain fatty acids.	• before physical exercise: increase muscle glycogen • during exercise: preventing shortage of muscle and liver glycogen • after physical exercise: re-plenish muscle glycogen
Products with a high protein content • concentrated proteins, (or mixture amino acids) • branched-chain amino acids • specific amino acids • creatine, carosine and other peptides	• supplying amino acids for protein synthesis • anabolic stimulus; energy supply: preventing over training • specific action • specific action
Supplements providing micronu-trients • vitamins, minerals, polyvitamin and/or polymineral substances • vitamin and/or non-vitamin antioxidants • iron minerals or other products with a high iron content	• preventing or treating vitamin and mineral deficiency • preventing the negative effects of free radicals • sideropenic anemia or depletion of iron stores
Bi-carbonate and other alkaline substances	• anti-acid effect
natural supplments (royal jelly, pollen, ginseng, eleutherococcus, brewer's yeast, various herbal products)	• various effects

is really absorbed in the intestine, for example.

In general, it is possible to say that the human being was not pro-grammed to tolerate the daily training loads which are necessary to reach and maintain top physical performance. Practicing ten times a week for many months a year, as most professional players gener-ally do, can cause considerable losses of iron and - in case of a tra-ditional diet - the digestive apparatus of some athletes is not able to absorb the suitable amount of iron to replace the loss.

Therefore, there are several reasons to use ready-made dietary supplements (canned, powder or tablets). The important thing is to ingest what one really needs.

However, it is fundamental to clearly identify the limit between correctly supplementing the diet and doping; actually, those who regularly practice heavy physical exercise are more likely to experi-ence testosterone deficiencies, but this does not mean they are allowed to take it in. The following paragraph is mainly focused on how athletes can avoid exceeding this critical limit.

DIFFERENT KINDS OF DIETARY SUPPLEMENTS
In the table on page 74 you will find a classification of the main dietary supplements commonly used in sport. Like many other clas-sifications it is absolutely disputable; as a matter of fact, I cannot exclude that the constant advance in scientific research will provide fresh knowledge in the field of dietology and new information as to dietary supplements in the next few years.

In the third chapter we discussed the benefits deriving from the ingestion of vitamin and mineral supplements and other antioxidant products, while the second chapter has clearly explained the impor-tance of drinking suitable beverages to replace the loss of fluids.

The next paragraphs will focus the attention on all the other dietary supplements, whose importance has already been pointed out on other occasions throughout the book.

Carbohydrates and other energy suppliers
In the first and second chapters we clearly explained that soccer players considerably benefit by carbohydrate supply, both foods and supplements. The importance and the effects of carbohydrate intake are strictly connected to the situation and the moment when these substances are ingested. In short, it is possible to suggest that:

- taking carbohydrates before the competition enhances the production of glycogen in muscles;
- carbohydrate intake during the match helps to prevent muscle glycogen depletion, which would seriously impair physical efficiency, and shortage of liver glycogen, which would lower glycemia levels,;
- carbohydrate supply after the competition can increase muscle glycogen stores; moreover, it is of critical importance if the next match is only a few days away.

A soccer player's diet before and after the match should provide suitable amounts of carbohydrates. Therefore, pasta, bread, potatoes, fruit, cookies and cakes, without cream or custard, are highly recommended. Immediately before, during and after the competition, on the contrary, it is very important for athletes to ingest easily digestible carbohydrates, in particular:

- *fructose:* compared to the other simple sugars providing the same calorie supply, it takes a much shorter time to pass through the stomach; moreover, it is absorbed more gradually and slowly in the intestine, thus avoiding variations in glycemia and insulinemia levels; this is extremely important in the minutes immediately before the competition;
- *glucose and sucrose:* they are particularly recommended immediately after the match, when players need to re-plenish muscle glycogen stores; actually, the increase in blood insulin concentration is a favorable factor in this case, since glucose molecules can easily penetrate the membrane of muscle fibers, thus helping glycogen synthesis;
- *maltodextrins:* they pass much more rapidly through the stomach than glucose and sucrose; although they consist of several linked glucose molecules, most of these bonds are quickly broken down in the intestine, so that when maltodextrins are dissolved in water, glucose molecules begin to flow into the bloodstream a very short time later.

These carbohydrates are usually dissolved in water, rather than ingested in tablets, that is in a solution which already provides part of the mineral salts players abundantly lose while sweating such as sodium, chlorine, magnesium and potassium. For this reason, one single beverage can be used to provide both fluid, water and salt, and energy in the form of carbohydrate supply. Remember that if sugar intake, during the competition or immediately before, is aimed not only at feeding energy stores but also at helping re-hydration, by drawing water in the blood, players had better take a mixture of different sugars, fructose and maltodextrins are particu-larly effective from this point of view, instead of one single variety, either glucose or fructose for instance.

Branched-chain amino acids

Branched-chain amino acids, that is valine, leucine and isoleucine, are substances of vital importance for the body. This means that the human being necessarily needs to introduce these elements - together with the six other essential amino acids - to defend his body and prevent illnesses. A healthy person who does not practice any kind of physical exercise needs about 5.4 grams of branched-chain amino acids every day: 1.6 grams of valine, 2.4 grams of leucine and 1.4 grams of isoleucine.

The human being needs to constantly provide his body with these simple but vital substances of which proteins are made; and all the proteins of food actually contain branched-chain amino acids in different percentages: from 15% (proteins of bread and pasta) to more than 22% (proteins of some cheeses).

Considering that the typical diet can provide more than 1.2 grams of proteins a day, sometimes even 1.5 grams, per every kilo-gram of body weight, it is easy to understand that daily branched-chain amino acid intake is very likely to exceed 15 grams, or even 20 grams in some cases.

It is important to underline that physical exercise increases the need for proteins in general, however, 1.5 grams a day are undoubt-edly enough for those who train hard, and for branched-chain amino acids in particular.

Some suggest that players should satisfy the increased need for essential amino acids with foods exclusively, without applying to dietary supplements; but, as was explained before, when branched-chain amino acids are provided by the proteins of food, (meat, cheese, milk, eggs...) at the same time the body inevitably receives large amounts of saturated fats, which are extremely harmful to the health, and a huge quantity of other unnecessary amino acids, dif-ferent from branched-chain amino acids.

The daily dose of branched-chain amino acids usually recommended to athletes is 0.1-0.2 grams per every kilogram of body weight, (that is 7.5-15 grams if the body weight is 75 kilograms). Higher amounts are generally prescribed in case of very strenuous exercise. This means that some 200 to 400 grams of extra meat should be included in the usual diet and, consequently, this would provide a surplus of non-branched-chain amino acids, 30 to 60 grams in excess, hundreds of calories and ten grams of saturated fats.

This is the reason why many athletes prefer to supplement their diet with the nutrients they really need, and therefore take branched-chain amino acid supplements.

Moreover, it is important to remember that branched-chain amino acids do not store up in the body as many supplements do, thus causing various disorders. Actually, in the human body there are some special enzymes which immediately attack the single amino acid molecules, either to link them together to form new protein molecules or to destroy them when no proteins are needed in the body. In practice, our body has no amino acid stores.

In short, branched-chain amino acids are absolutely harmless to our health in the amounts usually recommended to athletes - about 0.1-0.2 grams per every kilogram of the body weight (which means 7.5 to 15 grams if the body weight is 75 kilograms); serious disorders would result from the ingestion of huge doses, amounting to hundreds of grams of molecules every day.

However, as explained in the box on page 80, it is proven that in case of very intense physical training, the regular ingestion of branched-chain amino acids helps the athlete tolerate training loads to a greater extent, so that the over-training index always lies within a certain range: in short, also after the most strenuous training sessions, the anabolic process, (the synthesis of new proteins and the reconstruction of the proteins broken down during exercise) tends to prevail over the catabolic mechanism (the metabolic breakdown of large protein molecules). In a few words, branched-chain amino acids help athletes to recover much more rapidly from the fatigue and the efforts experienced while practicing or playing matches. Finally, players are less vulnerable to muscular disorders.

Creatine

Creatine is a peptide, a small protein molecule occurring in many body tissues, but mainly concentrated in muscle tissue (95%, at least). Muscle creatine concentration, however, can vary from one person to another and, in the same person, it strictly depends on the situation: from a maximum of 4.6 grams per every kilogram of muscle it can drop to a minimum of 3 grams or a little more. Compared to all the other small molecules occurring in muscle tissue, creatine is the element with the highest concentration: a male whose body weight is about 70 kilograms is supposed to have 80 to 130 grams of creatine in his muscles.

The human body is able to synthesize creatine by itself: actually, this compound is synthesized in the liver and in the kidneys from three amino acids - arginine, glycine and methionine. After passing through the liver and the kidneys, it enters the bloodstream and is conveyed to the muscles. In many cases the amount of substance produced in the body cannot replace the daily loss of creatine, which is considerably enhanced by strenuous physical exercise. Fortunately, creatine can be introduced in the body through the diet: this substance mostly occurs in meat and its concentration strictly depends on how the food is cooked. This dose of creatine, usually less than 1 gram a day and much more when much meat is ingested, is easily absorbed in the intestine and conveyed to the muscles. 4.6 grams of creatine per every kilogram of muscle tissue appears to be the maximum concentration in the human being. Muscle creatine concentration is undoubtedly lower in vegetarians and in those who eat little meat, but also in case of severe loss or reduced production of creatine by the liver and the kidneys.

Muscle creatine concentration inevitably influences muscle efficiency (see the box on page 82). Muscular resistance in spurts is seriously impaired, the recovery after a sprint is increasingly difficult and lactic acid easily poisons muscle tissue. In this case, the athlete can considerably benefit from creatine intake, combined with carnosine, if necessary.

On the contrary, those who already have maximum creatine concentrations (4.6 grams per every kilogram of muscle), cannot improve their performance by using creatine supplements. Muscle biopsy, the removal of a very small portion of muscle tissue, would be the ideal method to diagnose whether the athlete needs to take creatine or not; but this is an impracticable solution. When a player begins to use creatine supplements, within a short time he should be able to realize whether he really benefits from this substance or not: in the positive case, not only is the physical performance enhanced, but there is also an increase in the body weight, this is just a temporary variation in most cases.

When creatine was initially used as a dietary supplement in sport, (Swedish athletes were the first to use it, immediately followed by British sprinters) athletes were usually administered incredibly large doses: nearly 30 grams a day. Today, the amounts have been reduced considerably: 0.10-0.15 grams per every kilogram of the body weight, that is 7 to 10.5 grams a day if the body weight is 70 kilograms, for the first three or four days. Then, the athlete can use the so-called maintenance dose, corresponding to one third of the initial amount, that is about 3 grams.

Like the creatine of foods, the creatine in tablets or powder can also easily reach muscle tissue. It is useless to take phosphocreatine orally for two main reasons: first of all, it would not be absorbed and

PHYSICAL EXERCISE, CATABOLISM, ANABOLISM AND BRANCHED-CHAIN AMINO ACIDS

In order to understand one of the most important roles of branched-chain amino acids in sport, it is first of all necessary to tell something - even though in very simple terms - about catabolism and anabolism. During physical exercise (training session or competition) the body has a sort of catabolic attitude, which means it tends to break down big molecules into much smaller molecules so as to easily use them. When glycogen molecules are broken down, they release very small glucose molecules, which are a major source of energy both in aerobic process, where glucose combine with oxygen, and in lactic-acid anaerobic mechanism, where lactic acids build up from glucose. Proteins are broken down to release the elementary molecules they are made up of: amino acids. Some of them are burnt, while others are synthesized through a series of biochemical reactions.

By simple blood drawing during physical exercise, it is possible to observe that the body experiences an increase in catabolic hormones, cortical, in particular, and a drop in anabolic hormones, testosterone, for instance.

After the training session (not immediately after, but within a period of time which directly depends on the intensity of the physical performance: the harder the training session, the longer the period) the body has, or should have, a sort of anabolic behavior by which it builds up new molecules. These molecules are of critical importance in order to replace the destructive processes occurring while practicing physical exercise and to help the body adapt to the new changes and conditions in relation to the goals set for that specific training session. But remember that the body can undergo changes only if physical exercise has been performed properly.

When the training session is aimed at improving speed skills, for example, one of the main goals is to increase the muscular mass, which is possible only if the muscle tissue synthesizes new protein molecules, especially those - like actin and myosin - which interact to bring about muscle contraction. When physical exercise is aimed at improving aerobic power, on the contrary, the main goal for the body is to stimulate the synthesis of some specific enzymes in the mitochondrions.

However, when the training session is particularly heavy the catabolic process can prevail over the anabolic one in the hours immediately after and, in some cases, even for several days. In athletes who regularly practice strenuous exercise and recover little, the level of catabolic hormones is constantly high, while that of anabolic hormones is steadily low. Therefore, the ratio between testosterone concentration and cortisol concentration is always very low. In this situation, it is very difficult for the body to recover the original condition, the physical performance is very poor and training does not improve the athlete's physical condition, and in some cases even worsens it.

But what role do amino acids play in this complex situation?

It is proven that regular amino acid intake helps players practice strenuously and constantly, preventing any drop in anabolic hormones and any increase in catabolic hormone concentration. In short, they can recover much more easily from the fatigue of hard practice, which considerably wears out their body.

THE THREE ADVANTAGES OF CREATINE IN SOCCER

In soccer, and in all the other sport disciplines where periods of hard work usually alternate with periods of little physical activity, like basketball, tennis, volleyball, squash, rugby and hockey, creatine intake could be particularly helpful for three main reasons.

1. Creatine is an additional reserve of energy which can be used immediately; muscles can use one single source of direct energy, one specific 'fuel' better known as ATP; but muscle ATP concentration cannot exceed certain limits, that is the amount which is burnt to perform very few light movements. However, 60 to 90% of creatine occur in muscle fiber in the form of phosphocreatine, a molecule providing the energy immediately used to yield new ATP as soon as existing ATP stores wear out. From this point of view, creatine acts as a 'fuel supply' for prompt use. When an athlete has to sprint 25 meters, he first uses the energy provided by ATP and then the energy drawn from phosphocreatine. Many athletes have low creatine concentrations, less than 4.6 grams per every kilogram of muscle tissue, and therefore little phosphocreatine: this mean that their supply of reserve energy is very reduced.

2. Creatine helps to repay oxygen debt more rapidly, thus accelerating physical recovery. In the short interval between one physical effort and the next immediately after a sprint, for instance, the body needs to repay the oxygen debt resulting from the previous effort. In soccer, this debt needs to be paid in a very short time. This is possible thanks to the mechanism by which fats and sugars are burnt out in the mitochondrions, inside muscular fiber, so as to provide energy. But only creatine can act as a carrier molecule transporting this energy out of the mitochondrions: creatine enters the mitochondrion, charges with energy, thus becoming phosphocreatine, leaves the mitochondrion, releases energy, it turns into creatine again, enters the mitochondrion once again and so on. In soccer and in all the other 'intermittent' sport disciplines, the prompt recovery between two consecutive physical efforts strictly depends on the training level and especially on a large supply of creatine in muscles.

3. Creatine prevents some of the undesirable side effects of lactic acid. In soccer, lactic acid constantly builds up in muscle fiber. When acidity grows muscle fiber experiences a sort of 'crisis'; acidity is partly defeated by special 'buffers': they include some particular peptides among which creatine plays a role of critical importance. From this point of view, however, carnosine, another peptide usually occurring in meat, is still more important and an increase in muscle carnosine concentration would be particularly helpful in this sense. Carnosine and creatine work synergically, so that when creatine is combined with carnosine, it can lower the acidity of muscle fiber during the match, thus delaying the onset of muscular fatigue.

secondly, creatine is easily changed into phosphocreatine in the body, except in periods of greatest physical effort.

Creatine intake should be suspended for one week every month or two, especially in the periods of light training or when no match is going to be played. Players can also avoid taking creatine when they do not practice, for instance both during the pauses in the soccer season and while on vacation.

Some believe that athletes should ingest creatine exclusively by eating meat, without applying to dietary supplements, exactly like branched-chain amino acids. These persons do not realize that it would be necessary to eat 2 kilograms of meat to introduce 9 grams of creatine every day, which means absorbing extra calories and fat!

Moreover, creatine is particularly expensive. Therefore, I would suggest that those who are not accustomed to strenuous exercise had better begin by practicing more and harder to improve their physical efficiency: it is undoubtedly much cheaper, at least! Furthermore, we have previously underlined that those who practice regularly, professional players in particular, are more likely to lose great amounts of creatine, and therefore need this substance most. However, though most players could really benefit from creatine intake, the choice for this particular substance in amateur soccer is often prohibited by the high costs.

The amateur player could choose to take creatine only before very important matches, either for the single player or for the whole team. He should start 6 days before the competition with different daily doses - 9 grams of creatine for the first two days and 3 grams the four other days. Without spending much money even those who usually have low creatine concentrations can easily find the solution to approach optimum levels.

Glutamine and other small protein molecules

In the last few years, sport dietitians have focused their attention on a group of small protein or amino acid molecules; some of these substances have not proven so effective as they were thought to be, while others appear to be absolutely helpful. Apart from branched-chain amino acids and creatine, the interest of researchers was mainly concentrated on three particular molecules: glutamine, carnitine and carnosine.

Glutamine: Glutamine is a non-essential amino acid, which means that it can be synthesized from other molecules directly by the liver. The real problem is the speed at which it can be synthesized in relation to the daily needs of every single athlete, which are undoubtedly higher in case of strenuous and sustained exercise. Moreover, most of the glutamine taken orally is 'captured' by the cells of the lining membrane of the intestine. Several researches have shown that shortage of glutamine is one of the causes of over-training and increased vulnerability to infection - two conditions which soccer players really fear. Furthermore, not only does exogenous glutamine supply enhance blood buffer's action, while carnitine and carnosine's plugging action takes place in fibers, but it also increases fat consumption. Glutamine can be synthesized from branched-chain amino acids, whose intake is particularly useful also from this point of view.

Carnitine: In the 1982 World Cup great attention was turned to carnitine, the peptide that was supposed to help the Italian team win the World Championship. In practice, carnitine is the molecule which helps to 'burn' fats, since it carries fragments of fatty substances into the mitochondrion. In the past, exogenous carnitine supply was supposed to increase fat consumption in the unit of time. But lately, several studies have denied that it is possible and that carnitine intake can somehow improve the athlete's performance. However, we should remember that the human body is able to synthesize sufficient amounts of creatine. Moreover, most energy in soccer is drawn from carbohydrate consumption and just a very little percentage derives from fat breakdown.

Carnosine: Like creatine, carnosine is a very small protein molecule which acts as a buffer 'plugging' the negative effects (acidity) of lactic acid in muscle fibers. The higher the concentration of carnosine buffers in fiber tissue, the larger the amount of lactic acid produced in this tissue, and, therefore, the greater the quantity of energy produced by the lactic-acid anaerobic mechanism, before reaching the acidity level - the so-called critical pH - finally impairing the fiber. Carnosine usually occurs in meat and - like creatine - it seems that the amount synthesized in the body is not enough to satisfy the human needs.

Several researches have been carried out on the real benefits deriving from the intake of amino acid molecules in sport - both essential and non-essential amino acids, also including the most atypical elements such as taurine, for instance. Researchers are now focusing their attention on a group of other peptide molecules, and in the near future, they will probably offer new important information definitely piercing through the secrets of the world of proteins.

Iron and the athlete's anemia

Soccer players are very likely to develop the so-called athlete's anemia - that is iron-deficiency anemia - even though they are much less vulnerable than long-distance runners, triathlon athletes, cyclists, and cross-country skiers. The athlete feels weary and particularly weak, his physical efficiency is considerably impaired so that he can hardly tolerate strenuous effort, recovers much more slowly than usual, and often suffers muscular pain.

Iron-deficiency anemia is due to the fact that the body loses more iron than it absorbs. Actually, frequent and sustained physical practice considerably enhances the loss of iron in sweat, urine and feces, while iron is much more difficult to absorb in the intestine (Arcelli, Fiorella, Iacoponi and De Rocco, 1995). Female soccer players are more vulnerable than men; in either case, those who have a predisposition to this disease and have already suffered once in their lives are more likely to relapse, unless they change their habits, dietary habits in particular.

However, iron is commonly difficult to absorb. The iron of vegetable foods, or non-heme iron, - of parsley, spinach, cocoa and brewer's yeast, for instance - is absorbed in very low percentages: less than 10% at best, or even less than 3% in some cases; that of animal nutriments like meat, giblets and fish, ferroheme, is absorbed up to 30% only in the most favorable situations. In addition, some particular substances occurring in foods: phytates, phosphates, sulfates, oxalates, carbonates, wine, tea or coffee tannins, milk and egg

THE 10 RULES TO
PROPERLY SUPPLEMENT ONE'S DIET

1. Soccer players can really benefit from the use of a few dietary supplements.

2. Before and during the competition players should drink special beverages providing small amounts of sugar and salt; these drinks are sometimes also very helpful after the match.

3. Branched-chain amino acid intake can be particularly important since it helps players to recover from physical exercise in training sessions and matches.

4. In some cases, exogenous creatine intake increases the reserve of prompt-use energy, helps players recover more rapidly after every physical effort, after a sprint, for instance, and prevents the undesirable side effects of lactic acid.

5. Carnosine intake also helps to prevent the negative effects of lactic acid.

6. Glutamine intake can enhance the athlete's resistance to infection, which sometimes lowers in cases of particularly strenuous physical exercise.

7. Carnitine appears to be useless for soccer players.

8. Those who are more vulnerable to the athlete's anemia, due to iron deficiency, should combine ferroheme intake, commonly occurring in meat and liver, with vitamin C intake, avoiding any other nutriment or drink for up to two hours earlier and two hours later.

9. Some vitamin molecules, vitamin C, vitamin E and beta-carotene or provitamin A, and some minerals - in addition to other substances occurring in fruit and vegetables defend the body from the undesirable side effects of free radicals.

10. As far as natural supplements are concerned, professional athletes should avoid taking herbal substances, since anti-doping tests could prove positive in some cases.

proteins..., hinder iron absorption, while vitamin C helps it.

The diet suggested by Tredici-Iacoponi-Arcelli (Arcelli, 1990) can help those who are more vulnerable to the so-called athlete's anemia to prevent iron deficiency. This particular diet combines the ingestion of ferroheme, that is beef steak, liver or any other variety of meat, with vitamin C intake, far from any other kind of nutriments.

In some cases, it is much more effective than mineral iron supplements.

Bicarbonate and other alkaline substances

Bicarbonate - the common white soluble compound generally used to relieve gastric disorders, to whiten teeth or to cook some cakes - is a typically alkaline substance. For this reason it can prevent some of the negative effects resulting from the production of lactic acid in muscles. As a matter of fact, the consequent increase in hydrogen ion concentration acts at different levels, for example by inactivating phosphofructokinase, an enzyme of vital importance in the lactic-acid anaerobic energy mechanism.

In particular, in a situation where the muscle fiber attains critical acidity levels, the so-called critical pH, that is the minimum pH level it can tolerate: it is lower in glycolytic fast-conducting fibers and higher in slow-conducting ones, the fiber is completely impaired.

It is important to underline that bicarbonate does not penetrate muscle fiber; but, if during physical exercise bicarbonate concentration is highest in the blood and in muscle extracellular fluid, it is much easier for the fiber to release hydrogen ions which are immediately inactivated by special buffers.

Therefore, muscle fibers can supply a larger amount of energy through the lactic-acid mechanism before attaining critical pH levels. This is why many believe that athletes benefit most in the disciplines where the lactic-acid component is particularly high.

Excessive exogenous bicarbonate intake, dietitians usually recommend a dose of 0.3 grams per every kilogram of the body weight, which means a little more than 20 grams if the body weight is 70 kilograms, often causes undesirable side effects especially affecting the digestive system, like nausea, vomiting and diarrhea.

In addition, the benefits on the physical performance - supposing that they really exist, but some researchers are not sure they really do - need to be found in those disciplines where large amounts of lactic acid build up in muscle fibers, for instance the disciplines involving maximum effort performed in a very limited period of time varying from seconds to a very few minutes, like in running 400 and 800 meters or swimming 100 and 200 meters.

For this reason, dietitians do not usually recommend bicarbonate supplements in soccer. Even though the lactic-acid anaerobic mechanism, causing lactic-acid to build up in muscles, is undoubtedly important in soccer, (Arcelli and Ferretti, 1993; Arcelli, 1995) lactic acid concentrations are never so high as in the above-mentioned sport disciplines.

In the meantime, some researchers are turning their attention to studying the effects of other alkaline substances, starting from sodium citrate, in sport, since they appear to be much more effective than bicarbonate and cause fewer undesirable side effects.

'Natural' supplements

In the last few years, great attention - both in sport and in the world in general - has been turned to 'natural' products, since they are supposed to be much healthier than 'artificial' substances produced by man. But this belief is completely wrong, since poisonous or even deadly substances also exist in nature.

Some of the most commonly known natural supplements were already used in the past. Brewer's yeast, for instance, provides vitamin B, iron, cobalt and protein. Cornseed oil, which is produced starting from the most precious part of the wheat grain: the seed, supplies vitamin E and various substances having antioxidant properties, defeating free radicals, in addition to unsaturated fatty acids, polychosanoles and other molecules. Royal jelly, the substance produced by worker bees which changes a larva into a queen bee, provides vitamins, proteins and other substances - (some of which have not been completely identified) - are present in minimum quantities, but are sometimes of critical importance. This product is actually supposed to prevent several disorders and to help people to recover from some particular diseases. In the same way, pollen - the fine, usually yellow, powder formed in flowers and then transformed by bees - is thought to have special healing properties.

As far as herbal products are concerned, they can sometimes be good for amateur athletes, while professional players should avoid these kinds of substances, especially because anti-doping tests are very likely to prove positive in many cases. Also, while the label on the packaging of the product clearly shows its content we cannot be completely sure of the amount and of the quality of the substances it contains

At the 1988 Olympic Games in Seoul, for instance, the British sprinter Linford Christie tested positive for one particular kind of ginseng and he was not disqualified only because he could prove his innocence; he had drunk a cup of herb tea which was commonly offered at the Olympic village. Another Italian athlete, Antonella Bevilacqua, had serious problems before the 1996 Olympic Games in Atlanta because she had not been able to understand that the Chinese word 'mahuang', appearing on the packaging of the herbal product she commonly used, meant Ephedra, from which ephedrine, a well-know forbidden stimulant, is drawn. Among all the different herbal products on the market, ginseng and eleutherococcus are, or have been, particularly successful in sport.

Appendix

MACRONUTRIENTS, MICRONUTRIENTS AND FIBERS
This first part of the appendix specifically focuses the attention on macronutrients (carbohydrates, proteins and fats), micronutrients (vitamins and minerals) and fibers.

Carbohydrates
Carbohydrates are also called glucides, but this term is quite outdated; carbohydrates exist in different forms and therefore have different features, in particular:
- **monosaccharides** are the simplest form of carbohydrate, consisting of one simple sugar molecule; they include glucose, or dextrose, and fructose;
- **disaccharides** consist of two carbohydrate molecules and include sucrose (common table sugar), and lactose (milk sugar;) both monosaccharides and disaccharides are easily soluble in water and for this reason they are also known as water-soluble sugars or simply sugars;
- very few sugar molecules form an **oligosaccharide**; oligosaccharides also include maltodextrins which are made up of short - or middle-length chains of glucose molecules linked together;
- a chain of disaccharides forms a **polysaccharide**, like starch, occurring in cereals and potatoes, or glycogen, present in the liver and in muscles.

Properties: they are mainly used to provide energy; the carbohydrates of foods are broken down into small sugar molecules during the digestive process so that they can be assimilated into the blood stream while they are in the intestine. Then, they are transported to the liver and to the muscle tissue, where glycogen builds up through continuous processes of synthesis. However, sugar molecules can also be converted to fat molecules stored up in the cells, adipocytes, acting as a real reserve of fat.

Origin: they have a vegetable origin in most cases; the most commonly used nutriments with a high carbohydrate content include the foods deriving from wheat, bread and pasta, or corn, polenta, rice, legumes, fruit; milk contains about 5% of lactose; honey more than 80% of sugar, fructose, glucose and sucrose in lower percentages; sucrose accounts for 99% of common table sugar.

The differences between the various carbohydrates: water-soluble sugars, monosaccharides and disaccharides, are supposed to take a very short time to be assimilated into the blood stream, while starch is assimilated much more slowly. But this is not always true, since some particularly starchy foods, new potatoes for instance, cause blood glucose concentration to suddenly grow, while fructose, which is a monosaccharide, is usually absorbed quite slowly. The reality is practically more complex than one would think.

The table on page 93 shows the carbohydrate content, total, insoluble and soluble, of the main nutriments.

Proteins

Proteins, or proteins, are long chains of several hundred elementary molecules - amino acids - linked together. The digestive process breaks down these chemical bonds, thus breaking down the protein into hundreds of amino acids which are absorbed in the intestine and assimilated into the blood stream.

Properties: The body needs these nutrients to build up new protein molecules; actually, apart from water, muscles mainly consist of proteins; these proteins are synthesized in the body by using the amino acids present in the proteins of foods. For this reason, it is possible to say that all the proteins occurring in the body are constantly renewed and repaired at a speed which varies from one case to another. Therefore, the body of an adult also needs to be provided with a suitable daily amount of proteins to accomplish this peculiar task, a sort of 'maintenance' of the body.

Origin: They can have either a vegetable or an animal origin. However, animal proteins are usually the best from the biological point of view, since they contain all the different amino acids in more similar proportions to what the body really needs to produce its own proteins. Remember that some 22 different kinds of amino acids are involved: most of them are non essential which means that the body can synthesize them, while the essential amino acids, cannot be synthesized by the liver and must be provided ready-made in the proteins of the diet. Vegetable proteins often lack one or more essential amino acids so that they provide a lower amount than the body really needs. However, combining two different vegetable proteins, for instance the protein of cereals and that of legumes, sometimes enhances their total biological value, since one protein is very likely to provide the amino acids which are missing in another protein, and vice versa.

Essential amino acids: In alphabetical order the eight essential amino acids are: isoleucine, leucine, lysine, methionine, phenylalanine, threonine, tryptophan and valine; three of them - isoleucine, leucine and valine - are branched-chain amino acids. Tyrosine and cysteine are sometimes included in this category: but they should be defined as 'complementary' amino acids, since in case of need, that is when the diet does not provide the suitable amount, tyrosine can be synthesized from phenylalanine and cysteine from methionine. Histidine is also considered an essential amino acid in children. The other amino acids which are neither 'essential' nor 'complementary' include: alanine, aspartic acid, glutamic acid, arginine, glycine, proline and serine.

The foods providing proteins: Proteins account for 20% of meat, but the percentage varies from one kind of meat to another: 15% in fish; 18 to 33% of cheese and a little more than 3% of milk. The yolk contains water and very precious proteins, which can also be found in pasta (10 to 12%), bread (about 9%), and legumes (18 to 24%) of their dried weight. The table on page 94 shows the protein content of the most commonly used nutriments.

Daily need: A healthy adult male needs 0.8 to 1 gram of proteins per every kilogram of his body weight, which means 56 to 70 grams a day if his body weight is 70 kilograms. Young people, pregnant females or nursing mothers and athletes who build up muscle tissue usually need much larger amounts of proteins. In the period of heavy physical exercise, soccer players generally do not need more than 1.2 grams of proteins per every kilogram of their body weight.

Fats

Triglycerides are by far the commonest kind of fats and consist of an ester of glycerol combined with three fatty acid molecules. Other fats having much more complex structures include phosphofats,

The carbohydrate content of the main nutriments (per 100 grams)

*The **first column** refers to total carbohydrates, the **second** to insoluble glucides (starch), and the **third** to water-soluble carbohydrates.*

Food	Total	Insol.	Sol.	Food	Total	Insol.	Sol.
Pasta	77	74	3	Orange	7		7
Rice	81	80	1	Banana	20	3	17
Bread	62	61	1	Cherries	9		9
Bread sticks	75	72	3	Strawberries	6	tr	6
Whole meal cereals	70	70	tr	Apple	11		11
Light cookies	82	64	18	Walnuts	5	2	3
Wheat flour	70	68	2	Pear	12		12
Corn flour	74	73	1	Peach	15		15
Beans	45	39	6	Grapefruit	6		6
Peas	50	47	3	Plum	12		
Lean beef	0			Grapes	16		
Chicken	0			Butter	1		1
Lean Pork	1			Bacon fat	0		
Beef liver	6			Margarine	0		
Ham	0			Olive oil	0		
Cured ham	0			Beer	3		
Salami	0			Wine (10 ounces)	2		
Sole	0			Milk Chocolate	54		54
Codfish	0			Marmalade	55		55
Whole milk	4		4	Honey	84		84
Skim milk	5		5	Plain cake	63	28	35
Yogurt	0			Sugar	100		100
Eggs	1						
Cream cheese	3		3				
GruyEre cheese	0						
Mozzarella	5		5				
Parmasan cheese	0						
Ricotta cheese	0						
Cream	3		3				
Carrot	9		9				
Chicory	3		3				
Onion	5		5				
Fennel	2		2				
Fresh mushrooms	4	1	3				
Dried mushrooms	14	2	12				
Lettuce	2		2				
Potatoes	16	15	1				
Tomatoes	4		4				
Spinach	4		4				
Apricot	10		10				
Pinapple	13		13				

cerebrosides and so on.

Properties: they are mainly used to provide energy, or, still better, they are the most concentrated source of energy, since one gram of fat provides 9 kilo-calories, compared to 4 kilo-calories of carbohydrates and 5 kilo-calories of proteins, only 4 of which are useable.

Origin: both vegetable fats, like oil, and animal fats, such as butter and lard, exist; vegetable fats are supposed to be healthier and therefore should be preferred to animal fats. In any case, a varied Western diet usually includes too much fat.

The foods providing fats: butter, olive oil, seed oil, margarine and lard are almost completely made up of fats; fats account for about 50% of oily nuts (walnuts, hazelnuts, almonds, peanuts...); nearly 25% of cheese (but there are considerable differences from one variety to another) and about 3.6% of whole milk. Meat's fat content is extremely variable: it can be lower than 4% in lean meat and higher than 20% in particularly fatty kinds of meat. The table on page 137 shows the fat content of the main nutriments.

Daily need: a few grams of fats a day are usually enough; fats transport special fat-soluble vitamins, (vitamin A, D and E); moreover, the body needs to absorb approximately ten grams of particular vegetable fatty acids every day. Therefore, it is impossible to completely exclude these nutrients from the diet, although it is very important to reduce fat intake as much as possible.

Undesirable side effects: fat digestion is often particularly difficult for a number of people; in general, but especially for those whose blood cholesterol concentration - LDL concentration in particular - is very high, it is better to limit animal fat intake, apart from the fat of fish, which does not belong to the category to avoid. The diet of athletes in particular should include few fried or long cooked fatty substances.

Vitamins

Vitamins are very important nutrients the body cannot synthesize by itself, so they must be provided ready-made in the diet. Each vitamin plays different and specific roles in the body (see the table on page 98). Water-soluble vitamins, which can be dissolved in water, include: B1, B2, B6, B12, pantothenic acid, C, folic acid, H and PP; while fat-soluble vitamins, which can be dissolved in fat, are; A, D, E

The protein content of the main nutriments (per 100 grams)

Food	Protein (g)	Food	Protein (g)
Pasta	12	Fennel	0
Rice	7	Fresh mushrooms	5
Bread	8	Dried mushrooms	36
Bread sticks	11	Lettuce	1
Whole meal cereals	13	Potatoes	2
Light cookies	8.5	Tomatoes	1
Wheat flour	9	Spinach	3
Corn flour	8	Apricot	0
Beans	23	Pinapple	0
Peas	20	Orange	0
Lean beef	19	Banana	1
Chicken	16.5	Cherries	1
Lean Pork	20	Strawberries	1
Beef liver	20	Apple	0
Ham	21	Walnuts	19
Cured ham	18	Pear	0
Salami	36	Peach	1
Sole	16	Grapefruit	0
Codfish	13	Plum	0
Whole milk	3	Grapes	0
Skim milk	3	Butter	1
Yogurt	5	Bacon fat	0
Eggs	13	Margarine	1
Cream cheese	16	Olive oil	0
GruyEre cheese	31	Beer	0
Mozzarella	19	Wine (10 ounces)	0
Parmasan cheese	32	Milk Chocolate	10
Ricotta cheese	7	Marmalade	1
Cream	2	Honey	0
Carrot	1	Plain cake	0
Chicory	1	Sugar	0
Onion	1		

and K. Some diseases are due to vitamin deficiencies: scurvy, for instance, results from lack of vitamin C, while rickets, in children, and osteomalacia, in adults, are due to vitamin D deficiency. However, in order to enjoy full well-being it is fundamental to supply the body with a higher amount of vitamins, especially those having anti-oxidant properties; (refer to the paragraph '**Free radicals: how to fight them off**' on page 61) than the minimum quantity which is necessary to prevent deficiency diseases. Different foods contain vitamins in different concentrations.

Minerals

Minerals, as well as vitamins, occur in foods in different concentrations. The lack of one single mineral can bring about disease. Some particular minerals (selenium, manganese, copper and zinc) are important not only to prevent deficiency diseases, but also to defeat free radicals and therefore need to be supplied in higher concentrations. Some electrolytes (sodium, chlorine, potassium, calcium and magnesium) are abundantly lost in sweat, so that they must be replaced with suitable foods and drinks immediately after physical exercise. The table on page 100 shows the important roles these substances play in the body and the natural sources of the main minerals.

Fibers

Dietary fibers occur in vegetable foods. These substances are not digested in our body since the digestive system has no enzymes to digest them; therefore, they are passed on to the large intestine, where they add to the bulk of the feces to be voided. It would be completely wrong to consider them as useless waste, since they are extremely important for the efficiency of our body. As a matter of fact, various diseases have been blamed on lack of fiber in the diet and constipation is by far the most common among them.

There are differences between one fiber and another; however, they can be divided into:
- **insoluble fibers:** the most common is undoubtedly cellulose, occurring in all fruits and greens;
  - they also include: hemicellulose and lignin;
- **soluble fibers:** pectin occurs in all fruits, its concentration is particularly high in quince and citrus fruits, while other soluble

fibers like glucomannan and galactomannan, which can be found only in some particular vegetables, have special slimming properties, so that they are extremely recommended to those who need to lose weight.

Soluble fibers are very useful to keep the intestine perfectly efficient, while insoluble fibers regulate the absorption of the molecules resulting from the digestion of foods; in particular, they prevent glycemia levels, and, consequently, insulin concentration too, from suddenly increasing when too many simple carbohydrates are ingested at a time.

THE VARIOUS FOOD GROUPS

The most commonly used nutriments can be divided into seven main groups, each one including foods sharing similar features, which should be represented in the diet. In general, this classification helps people to immediately and clearly understand the nutrient content of one particular food and to easily identify the possible alternatives for that food.

Some believe that each food group should be included in the daily diet; but this is an extreme simplification, since proteins with a high biological value, for instance, can be provided by different foods belonging either to the group A or to the group B, or by a combination of nutriment's falling in groups C and D.

Carbohydrate content is particularly high in the foods of groups C and D, but also F and G, while dietary fibers mainly occur in the nutriments of groups C, F, G and D.

In reality, this classification is most useful when a person needs to choose between two different courses, when he wants to rapidly analyze the total food intake and when it is necessary to know how to replace one particular nutriment with another. Here are the seven food groups:

Group A: meat, eggs, fish. - It includes all the different varieties of meat, including liver, beef, pork, poultry, game as well as fish, shellfish and eggs. All these foods provide proteins with a high biological value, vitamins B1, B2, PP, B12 and iron ferroheme, the easiest form of iron to absorb.

Group B: milk, yogurt and cheese. - This group includes milk, (fresh, condensed, and evaporated) and dairy products, like yogurt

The fat content of the main nutriments, per 100 grams
The values refer to total fats (T), saturated (S), monounsaturated (M) and polyunsaturated fats (P).

Food	T	S	M	P	Food	T	S	M	P
Pasta	1		0.5	0.5	Potatoes				
Rice	1		0.5	0.5	Tomatoes				
Bread	.05		tr	tr	Spinach				
Bread sticks	1		0.5	0.5	Apricot				
Whole meal cereals	7	2	4.5	0.5	Pinapple				
Light cookies	2	0.5	1	0.5	Orange				
Wheat flour	1	tr	0.5	0.5	Banana				
Corn flour	3	tr	1.5	1.5	Cherries				
Beans	2	0.5	1	0.5	Strawberries				
Peas	3	0.5	1.5	1	Apple				
Lean beef	7	3	3	1	Walnuts	47	3	34	10
Chicken	6	2	2	2	Pear				
Lean Pork	16	5	10	1	Peach				
Beef liver	3	2	0.5	0.5	Grapefruit				
Ham	36	16	15	5	Plum				
Cured ham	45	20	20	5	Grapes				
Salami	34	16	15	3	Butter	83	60	21	2
Sole	2	1.5	0.5	tr	Bacon fat	98	48	38	9
Codfish	2	1	1	tr	Margarine	83	30	23	10
Whole milk	3	2	1	tr	Olive oil	99	17	72	10
Skim milk	0.2	0.1	0.1	tr	Beer				
Yogurt	5	3	2	tr	Wine (10 ounces)				
Eggs	11	5.5	4	1.5	Milk Chocolate	31	18	11	2
Cream cheese	21	15	5	1	Marmalade				
GruyEre cheese	31	19	10	2	Honey				
Mozzarella	26	17	8	1	Plain cake	10	4	5	1
Parmasan cheese	29	19	9	1	Sugar				
Ricotta cheese	21	15	5	1					
Cream	35	22		2					
Carrot									
Chicory									
Onion									
Fennel									
Fresh mushrooms									
Dried mushrooms	3								
Lettuce									

VITAMINS

Water-soluble vitamins	Main Sources	Roles	Daily need (non-athletes)
B1 Thiamine	Brewer's yeast, corn germs, cereals, peanuts, liver, fish, meat	It preserves nerve cells and heart muscle. It prevents beriberi.	1.5 to 3 mg occurring in 10 to 20 g of Brewer's yeast, 200 g of other foods.
B2 Riboflavin	Brewer's yeast, milk, liver, vegetables, fish, whole meal cereals, eggs.	It stimulates the maturation of lymphocytes T. It helps nutriments to release energy.	2 to 3 mg occurring in 50 g of brewer's yeast. 100 g of other foods.
B5 Pantothenic	Greens, meat, liver, eggs, kidney.	It is necessary for fat and sugar metabolism and for the synthesis of some hormones.	4 to 7 mg occurring in 100 g of liver and eggs, 400 g of other foods.
B6 Pyridoxine	Brewer's yeast, legumes, cereal germs, red meat, salmon.	It is fundamental in protein metabolism and is involved in the nervous and the immune systems.	3 to 10 mg occurring in 100 to 200 g of brewer's yeast, 500 g of other foods.
B12 Cyanocobalamin	Milk, liver, kidney, fish.	It helps the maturation of red cells. It is necessary for the nervous and the immune systems.	3 to 10 mg occurring in 20 to 30 g of liver and kidney, 100 g of fish, 100 g of milk.
C Asorbic-acid	Vegetables (peppers, in particular), fruit (especially citrus fruits), liver.	It enhances iron absorption. It has anti-oxidant properties. It strengthens collagen and the immune system. It prevents scurvy.	100g of oranges, 200 g of strawberries, 50 g of peppers, 250 g of liver. Increasing the dose up to 1 g is usually recommended.
Folic Acid	Brewer's yeast, rice, corn germs, fruit, greens, liver.	It helps the maturation of red cells and the synthesis of nucleic acids.	400 to 1 mg occurring in 200 g of liver, 400 g of other foods.
H Biotin	Milk, vegetables, kidney, eggs.	It is involved in fat and sugar metabolism.	Abundantly provided in the diet.
PP Niacin	Brewer's yeast, eggs, lean meat, liver, whole meal cereals.	It is involved in carbohydrate metabolism. It prevents pellagra.	20 mg occurring in 150 g of liver, 50 g of brewer's yeast, 300 g of other foods. Fat soluble.
A Retin	Milk, butter, cheese, vegetables, carrots, spinach, liver, fish liver oil, yolk.	It stimulates growth, It defends the skin, It prevents night blindness.	25000U.I. occurring in 800 g of yolk, 100 g of liver, 250 g of cheese, 300 g of carrots.
D Calciferol	Milk, fish, liver, eggs, prolonged exposition to sun radiation.	It strengthens teeth and bones, it promotes the absorption of calcium and phosphorus, it prevents rickets.	10 ug for children, 5 ug for adults occurring in 400 g of milk, 200 g of liver, 100 g of salmon, 50 g of eggs.
E Tocopheroll	Corn germs, vegetable oil.	It has anti-oxidant properties. It avoids excessive consumption of fat in tissues.	300 U.I. occurring in 30 g of corn germs, 3 g of vegetable oil - the dose can be increased up to 400 U.I.
K Menadinoe	Greens, vegetable oil, pork meat.	It is required for the formation of the enzyme thrombin. It helps healthy blood clotting.	Not established; suggestion: 10 ug occurring in 25 g of cauliflower, 100 g of liver.

Minerals

Mineral	Role in the Body	Natural Sources
Sodium	It regulates the volume of the body fluids, their basicity and their acidity.	Meat, fish, milk, cheese, bread, greens, nuts, kitchen salt.
Chlorine	Production of gastric juice, transport of carbon dioxide from tissues to the lungs and acid-base balance.	Kitchen salt, caned meat, smoked fish, shellfish, olives.
Potassium	It is responsible for the life cycle of the cells of both smooth and striated muscles and of the nervous tissue; it intervenes to maintain body water balance.	Meat, milk, fish, legumes, potatoes, cabbage, parsley, apricots, bananas, pinapple.
Calcium	It forms the hard framework of bones, teeth and nails; it intervenes in blood clotting and muscle motility.	Milk, cheese, eggs, dried legumes, greens.
Phosphorus	Formation of bones and teeth; it intervenes in the metabolism of proteins, fats and glucides as well as in energy processes; it is one of the main components of the cerebral tissue.	Milk, cheese, meat, poultry, fish, oats, lentils, artichokes, yeast, corn germs.
Magnesium	It is involved in the structure of muscle tissue and nerve bundles.	Whole meal cereals, greens, nuts.
Iron	It is one of the main components of hemoglobin, myoglobin and of the enzymes involved in different metabolisms.	Eggs, giblets, lean meat, legumes, whole meal cereals, greens, nuts.
Iodine	It is a component of thyroid hormones.	Sea fish, milk, eggs, sea salt, many vegetables.
Sulfur	It is a constituent of living compounds in tissues, cartilage and tendons.	Meat, eggs, legumes, garlic, onion.
Copper	It is involved in the synthesis of hemoglobin.	Meat, eggs, legumes, nuts, garlic, onion.
Zinc	It is a constituent of insulin.	Cereals, yeast, legumes, tomatoes, spinach, herrings.
Fluorine	It is one of the main components in the structure of bones and teeth.	Sea products, peas.
Manganese	It is involved in fat metabolism	Cereals, almonds, peas.

and cheeses. They supply proteins with a high biological value, such as vitamins B1 and B2 and calcium.

Group C: legumes. - It includes beans, lentils, chickpeas, peas, broad beans, soy beans and so on. These nutriments provide: proteins with a middle biological value. Their biological value is considerably enhanced if legumes are combined with foods belonging to the group D.

Group D: cereals and their by-products. - It includes: cereals, wheat, corn, rice, barley..., and their by-products like bread, bread sticks, crackers, pasta, polenta and so on. These foods provide: carbohydrates; vitamins B1, B2 and PP; proteins with a middle biological value (which are complementary to the proteins provided by legumes - group C); and dietary fibers (the amount strictly depends on their refining level).

Group E: oil and fats. - It includes: butter, olive oil, all the different kinds of seed oil, lard, margarine. From these foods the body mainly absorbs fats and, in some cases, vitamin or provitamin A, butter and olive oil, vitamin E, some varieties of oil, and essential fatty acids, oil, in particular.

Group F: vegetables and fruits (yellow, orange or green fruits). - The main nutriments belonging to this group are: carrots, apricots, yellow peaches, pumpkin, persimmons, plums, bananas, apples, pears, peppers, beets, cabbage, savoy cabbage, broccoli, cauliflower, endive and other kinds of green salad, spinach, zucchini, and string beans. They provide: vitamin A and/or carotene, that is provitamin A; dietary fibers; carbohydrates, the percentage varies from one nutriment to another: some fruits have maximum carbohydrate content while some greens have minimum carbohydrate concentrations; mineral salt, like phosphorus, magnesium and iron (non-heme).

Group G: tomatoes and citrus fruits. - This group includes: tomatoes, oranges, lemons, grapefruits, tangerines and also strawberries and kiwi fruits. They supply considerable amounts of vitamin C, which, also occurs in other vegetable foods, especially in some fruits and fresh greens.

The fiber content of various foods

The fiber content, soluble and insoluble fibers, of various nutriments, in grams per 100 grams of edible substance. (R) means raw vegetables; (B) means boiled vegetables and (C) refers to cooked vegetables.

	Soluble Fibers	Insoluble Fibers		Soluble Fibers	Insoluble Fibers
CEREALS AND BY-PRODUCTS			Aubergines (C)	2.3	1.2
			Potatoes (B)	0.9	0.7
			Peppers (R)	1.5	0.5
Light crackers	1.8	1.5	Tomatoes (R)	0.8	0.2
Bran crackers	6.2	0.9	Radish (R)	1.2	0.1
Wheat flour	1.0	1.5	Celery (R)	1.4	0.2
White bread	1.7	1.5	Spinach (B)	1.6	0.4
Whole meal bread	5.4	1.2	Savoy cabbage (R)	2.5	0.7
Cooked pasta	0.9	0.5	Zucchini (B)	1.0	0.4
Boiled rice	0.6	0.5			
LEGUMES			**SALAD**		
Cooked chickpeas	9.1	0.5	Belgian salad	1.0	0.2
Cooked beans	5.8	0.8	Endive	1.4	0.2
Cooked broad Beans	6.8	0.6	Lettuce	1.3	0.1
			Red radishes	2.4	0.6
Lentils	7.2	0.2	**FRUIT**		
			Apricots	0.8	0.7
VEGETABLES			Pineapple	0.8	0.2
			Oranges	1.0	0.6
Asparagus (B)	1.6	0.5	Bananas	1.2	0.6
Broccoli (B)	2.5	0.6	Cherries	0.8	0.5
Artichokes (B)	3.2	4.7	Watermelon	0.2	0.0
Carrots (R)	2.7	0.4	Figs	1.4	0.6
Carrots (B)	1.6	1.5	Strawberries	1.1	0.5
Cauliflower (B)	1.7	0.7	Kiwi fruits	1.4	1.8
Cabbage (R)	2.3	0.3	Tangerines	1.0	0.7
Cabbage (B)	2.0	0.7	Apples	1.4	0.6
Cucumbers (R)	0.5	0.2	Melon	0.6	0.2
Chicory (R)	2.4	1.2	Pears	2.3	0.6
Onion (R)	0.9	0.2	Peaches	1.4	0.9
Onion (B)	0.8	0.5	Grapefruits	1.0	0.0.
French beans (B)	2.1	0.9	Plums	0.8	6
Fennel (R)	2.0	0.3	Grapes	1.2	0.2

INTAKE AND LOSSES

Intake

The energy deriving from foods and drinks, that is the calorie intake, can be estimated on the basis of the amount of proteins, carbohydrates and fats occurring in the nutriments and beverages one has ingested; it is particularly easy to calculate these amounts when referring to the data concerning the content of various foods, as they clearly appear in the tables on page 98, 99 and 100, for instance. Moreover, it is important to remember that:

- each gram of proteins and carbohydrates provides 4 kilo-calories while
- each gram of fats yields 9 kilo-calories.

Also, don't forget that each gram of alcohol provides 7 kilo-calories.

It is also possible to refer to special tables, like that on page 107, which directly show the energy content of foodstuffs. Remember that, in reality, proteins, carbohydrates and fats usually supply slightly higher amounts of calories than those included in the table, one gram of fats, for instance, does not provide 9 kilo-calories on average, but 9.3. This is due to the fact that using round figures is much more practical and because the nutrients ingested are not assimilated completely, a part of them is usually lost.

Losses

In order to calculate the energy requirement of a person, that is the total amount of calories he needs, it is necessary to add two important components:

- his basic energy requirement at rest, that is the calories spent while at full rest, various hours after eating, in completely favorable weather conditions;

total energy requirement =	energy requirement at rest + energy requirement at work

Basic energy requirement, at rest

If a car spends no fuel at all while it is parked in the garage, the human body, on the contrary, inevitably spends calories also when it is at full rest. All the cells in the body consume energy to survive, the heart consumes energy to pump blood, the respiratory apparatus to breathe, the kidneys and all the various glands to work and so on.

There are several possible methods to calculate the basic energy requirement, which is also called 'basal metabolic rate' - BMR. The most practical, and sufficiently precise methods are undoubtedly the Harris and Benedict formulae, which help to measure the daily basic energy requirement expressed in kilo-calories per 24 hours:

- **for men:** 66.473 + 13.752 W + 5.003 H - 6.755 A
- **for female:** 655.096 + 9.563 W + 1.850 H - 4.676 A

In these formulae: W refers to the body weight expressed in kilo-grams, H to the height expressed in centimeters and A to the age expressed in years.

The daily basic energy requirement, that is the total amount of calories he would spend if he were at rest for 24 hours, of a 24-year-old soccer player - whose body weight is 72 kilograms and whose height is 178 centimeters - would be nearly 1800 kilo-calories (kcal), as it results from the following calculation:

13.752 x 72 (body weight in kg)	66.473 kcal +
	990.144 kcal +
5.003 x 178 (height in cm)	890.534 kcal -
6.755 x 24 (age in years)	162.120 kcal =
	1785.031 kcal

The basic energy requirement of the athlete in question amounts to about 1.24 kilo-calories per minute.

A 19-year-old female soccer player, whose body weight is 58 kilo-grams and whose height is 163 centimeters, is supposed to need a little more than 1400 kilo-calories per day:

9,563 x 58 (body weight in kg)	655.096 kcal +
1,850 x 163 (height in cm)	554.654 kcal +
	301.550 kcal -
4,676 x 19 (age in years)	88.844 kcal =
	1422.456 kcal

The basic energy requirement of this girl amounts to nearly one kilo-calorie per minute.

The energy requirement at work

The energy requirement while at work is extremely different from one person to another. As far as soccer players are concerned, their energy requirements strictly depend on whether they practice physical exercise or not.

However, apart from the expense of energy due to muscular work, both during physical exercise and while carrying out common daily activities, the energy requirement at work also results from two other important components:

- the energy requirement for thermoregulation, that is the energy used to maintain the internal body temperature at about 37 degrees centigrade;
- the energy requirement for the specific-dynamic action of foods, that is the energy spent by the body to carry out all the digestive and metabolic processes following the ingestion of foods.

Consequently:

Energy requirement at work = energy spent for thermoregulation
+ energy spent for the specific-dynamic action of foods
+ energy spent for muscular exercise

Thermoregulation, specific-dynamic action of foods, muscular work

It is extremely difficult to perfectly calculate all the different components of the energy requirement at work. The energy spent for the process of thermoregulation, for instance, strictly depends on the weather conditions in which the person lives. On its turn, the spe-

Energy value and water content of the main nutriments
(per 100 grams of edible substance)

Food	Calories kcal	Water	Food	Calories kcal	Water
Pasta	370	12	Orange	35	87
Rice	360	13	Banana	85	76
Bread	273	32	Cherries	41	86
Bread sticks	385	9	Strawberries	33	90
Whole meal cereals	391	8	Apple	46	85
Light cookies	351	5	Walnuts	690	10
Wheat flour	350	14	Pear	48	85
Corn flour	366	12	Peach	66	90
Beans	316	62	Grapefruit	25	91
Peas	340	75	Plum	50	87
Lean beef	90	72	Grapes	64	880
Chicken	165	68	Butter	755	15
Lean Pork	150	72	Bacon fat	852	2
Beef liver	140	70	Margarine	760	16
Ham	415	37	Olive oil	900	0
Cured ham	480	34	Beer	35	91
Salami	470	26	Wine (10 ounces)	78	89
Sole	84	80	Milk Chocolate	545	2
Codfish	84	81	Marmalade	230	30
Whole milk	62	87	Honey	302	18
Skim milk	34	90	Plain cake	368	20
Yogurt	60	87	Sugar	410	1
Eggs	155	74			
Cream cheese	247	57			
GruyEre cheese	420	32			
Mozzarella	340	60			
Parmasan cheese	395	30			
Ricotta cheese	235	65			
Cream	340	58			
Carrot	46	91			
Chicory	22	93			
Onion	27	92			
Fennel	8	93			
Fresh mushrooms	38	92			
Dried mushrooms	316	12			
Lettuce	12	94			
Potatoes	85	82			
Tomatoes	24	94			
Spinach	36	90			
Apricot	40	86			
Pineapple	52	87			

cific-dynamic action of foods inevitably varies according to the content of nutriments, it is about 28 to 30% for proteins, 2 to 8% for fats and 5 to 10% for carbohydrates.

In general, in order to simplify the question it is possible to fix a broad calorie requirement for thermoregulation, for the specific-dynamic action of foods and also for all the movements which are connected neither to sport training nor to work activities (speaking, moving one's eyes, moving from one place to another, dressing and many other movements everybody carries out in common daily life). This fixed calorie requirement amounts to: 650 kilo-calories for male soccer players and 550 kcal for female players.

The energy spent in work activities

In order to calculate the total amount of energy spent while carrying out work activities, although it is almost impossible to know the exact quantity, it is possible to refer to some particular tables - like the one below - in which the energy expense is expressed in kilo-calories per minute:

the kind of work	male (65 kg)	female (65 kg)
light (sedentary work involving light load)	1.5-3.0	1.2-2.8
average (standing work involving important commitment)	5.0-7.4	3.5-5.4
heavy (like masons or miners)	7.5-9.9	5.5-7.4

For instance, a male soccer player - who works as a designer 8 hours a day (480 minutes) and whose energy expense is about 1.5 kilo-calories per minute - daily spends: 1.5 kcal/min x 480 min = 720 kilo-calories for his work, for 5 days a week.

A female soccer player - who has a part-time job as a clerk and therefore stands 4 hours a day (240 minutes), and whose energy expense is about 2 kilo-calories per minute - spends: 2 kcal/min x 240 = 480 kilo-calories every working day.

The energy spent during the training session and the match

Several studies carried out on soccer players have shown that the goalkeeper spends about 4.5 to 5.3 kilo-calories per minute, while the energy expense of the other players varies from 5 to 19 kcal/min during the match. Moreover, the higher the general level of the whole team, the higher the energy expense of the players. As a matter of fact, minimum energy expense values usually refer to amateur players, while professional soccer players, especially those in the first division, usually spend most.

Therefore, a good amateur player, playing for the whole match (90 minutes) is supposed to spend slightly more than 1000 kilo-calories. A professional player generally spends more than 1500 kilo-calories, especially if he moves a lot while on the playing field. Female soccer players spend 20% less than men on average.

With the time of both the training session and the match being equal, the energy expense is most often lower during the training session than during the competition. According to Reilly, 1990, it is possible to assess the energy expense for each kind of physical exercise:

gymnastics and stretching, warm up and warm down	7.5 kcal/min
slow running	14.0 kcal/min
circuit training or weight-lifting	10.2 kcal/min
training to improve technical skills	10.8 kcal/min
match	16.2 kcal/min

By clearly recording the exact time spent on each kind of physical exercise, it is possible to approximately calculate the total amount of energy spent during a whole training session. Here is an example:

10 min stretch and mobility of the back: 7.5 kcal/min x 10 min	75 kcal
12 min slow running: 14 kcal/min x 12 min	168 kcal
20 min muscular training with weights: 10.2 kcal/min x 20 min	204 kcal
18 min technique: 10.8 kcal/min x 18 min	194 kcal
15 min match: 16.2 kcal/min x 15 min	243 kcal
06 min warm down: 7.5 kcal/min x 6 min	45 kcal
during a training session lasting one hour and 21 minutes the soccer player spends	**929kcal**

This total energy expense value refers to male soccer players and, since female athletes usually spend 20% less than men, their energy expense is about 745 kilo-calories during the same training session.

Total energy expense
If we consider the two soccer players, one male and one female, having the above-mentioned characteristics (weight, job...), it is possible to assess that during any common week day including not only their usual work activities but also the training session like that shown in the previous table, their total energy expense is approximately:

	male	female
thermoregulation, specific-dynamic action, etc.	650 kcal	550 kcal
work activity	720 kcal	480 kcal
training	929 kcal	745 kcal
	2299 kcal	1775 kcal

As far as the basic energy requirement is concerned, it can be calculated on the 24 hours. In this case, the male would spend 1785 kilo-calories at rest while the female would need 1422 kilo-calories at rest. Since it is necessary to deduct the working hours, 8 hours for the male and 4 hours for the female, and the hours spent practicing physical exercise (1 hour 21 minutes):
- the male soccer player's basic energy requirement is 1.24 kcal/min; it is calculated on the 24 hours (1440 minutes), minus 9 hours 21 minutes (561 minutes), and therefore amounts to: **1440 - 561 min x 1.24 kcal/min = 1090 kcal**
- the female soccer player's basic energy requirement is 1 kcal/min; it is calculated on the 24 hours (1440 minutes), minus 5 hours 21 minutes (321 minutes), and therefore amounts to: **1440 - 321 min x 1 kcal/min = 1119 kcal**

Therefore, during each working day including that particular training session, the total energy expense, resulting from the sum of the energy requirement at rest and the energy requirement at work, of the two athletes is respectively:

- male soccer player: basic energy requirement **1090 kcal** + energy requirement at work **2299 kcal** = the total energy expense is about **3389 kcal.**
- female soccer player: basic energy requirement **1119 kcal** + energy requirement at work **1775 kcal** = the total energy expense is about **2894 kcal.**

Anyway, it is particularly important to remember that all the values referring to the different energy requirements are just approximate figures, since it is extremely difficult to consider all the real factors influencing them.

GLOSSARY

Adipocytes (fat cells): any of the cells of adipose tissue, in which fats are stored.

Amino acids: they are the elementary constituents of proteins, both the proteins synthesized in our body and those of foods. Proteins are made up of various proportions of about 20 commonly occurring amino acids; eight of them are known as essential amino acids, since they cannot be synthesized by the liver and must therefore be provided ready-made in the proteins of the diet.

Anabolism: all the processes promoting the synthesis of new molecules in the body, like the synthesis of proteins, from amino acids, or of glucose, from simple sugar molecules.

Anti-doping test: medical examination especially carried out by sport leagues, or special bodies, in order to identify the athletes who use illegal substances.

Anti oxidants: important substances preventing the undesirable effects of free radicals; they include: endogenous anti oxidants, which means they are produced in the human body, and exogenous anti oxidants, which are introduced from outside through the diet.

Aspartates: aspartic acid salts, aspartic acid is one of the amino acids; some dietitians believe that aspartate intake helps to prevent muscular cramp.

Branched-chain amino acids: they belong to the group of essential amino acids, valine, leucine and isoleucine, and stimulate the synthesis of proteins.

Carbohydrates: the fundamental nutrients in the human diet; the simplest carbohydrates are the sugars - which consist of one or two linked molecules, monosaccharides and disacchrides, respectively, -

like fructose and sucrose (table sugar).

Carnitine: substance mainly occurring in meat and in human muscle tissue; it stimulates fat consumption.

Carnosine: substance occurring in meat and in human muscle tissue; it prevents the negative effects of lactic acid.

Catabolism: the processes promoting the breakdown of all the various molecules; the reference is often made to the catabolism of the proteins occurring in muscles, which therefore lose volume and strength.

Creatine: substance occurring in most meat and in human muscle tissue; shortage of creatine in muscles seriously impairs their efficiency.

Dehydration: considerable reduction in the total volume of water in the body; it often results from a considerable loss of water, because of severe sweating, for instance.

Diet: balanced mode of living; in common language, alimentary diet refers to the dietary regimen one usually follows for medical reasons or, in most cases, in order to lose weight; low calorie diet refers to a diet providing low amounts of calories.

Dietary fibers: substances, mainly carbohydrate molecules, usually occurring in vegetable foods which are not assimilated by the body during the digestive process, so that they are passed on to the large intestine and then excreted in the feces. They include: insoluble fibers, cellulose, hemicellulose and lignin, which especially stimulate the movements of the intestine; and soluble fibers, which are particularly important because they slow down sugar absorption.

Dietary supplements: nutrients supplementing the diet. These substances can be ingested as special beverages or dietary tablets.

Fatty acids: elementary molecules which most commonly occur, together with other molecules, as constituents of certain fats;

triglycerides, for instance, consist of one ester of glycerol and three molecules of fatty acids.

Free radicals: very reactive molecules which can seriously damage cell structure; they are the cause, or one of the main causes, of various disorders and diseases and also stimulate aging.

Fructose: a simple sugar occurring in fruits; it is a monosaccharide, which means it consists of one single elementary molecule; it is very similar to sucrose (table sugar), in terms of taste, sweetening value and calorie supply, but unlike sucrose, it does not bring about any increase in blood glucose and insulin concentrations. Moreover, it is digested in the stomach much more rapidly.

Glucose: simple sugar, widely occurring in nature; it is a monosaccharide, it consists of one single molecule, and combines with fructose to form sucrose (table sugar). Starch and glycogen are made up of long chains of linked glucose molecules. Glucose is the sugar occurring in the blood; it is also known as dextrose.

Glycemia: glucose concentration in the blood.

Glycogen: a carbohydrate which is very similar to starch, they both consist of long chains of linked glucose molecules, and which is present in the liver and in muscles.

HDLs: high density lipoproteins; particular substances occurring in the blood; they act to prevent heart infarction and various circulatory diseases. They are also defined as "artery scavengers," since they clean the lumen of these blood vessels.

High carbohydrate diet: diet providing larger amounts of carbohydrates than usual; it is generally recommended to increase glycogen concentration in the liver and in muscles.

Hyperglycemia: sudden increase in blood glucose concentration beyond normal levels.

Hyperlipidemia: excess of fat or fat-like substances in the blood.

Hypertonic solution: solution whose salt and sugar concentrations are higher than plasma's.

Hypoglycemia: sudden decrease in blood glucose concentration below normal levels; it can result from protracted fast, but also from excessive sucrose, common table sugar, or glucose intake. First of all, blood glucose concentration rapidly grows (hyperglycemia) but it immediately falls within a very short time, because of the intervention of insulin. This pathology is better known as reactive hypoglycemia, since it is brought about by the insulin's reaction to the previous increase.

Hypotonic solution: solution whose salt and sugar concentrations are lower than plasma's.

In perspiration: passive transudation of almost pure water from the surface of the body, without sweat glands being involved.

Insulin: a hormone produced in the pancreas and released into the bloodstream when there is an excess of glucose in the blood.

Insulinemia: blood insulin concentration.

Isoleucine: one of the three branched-chain amino acids.

Isotonic solution: solution whose salt and sugar concentrations are similar to blood's.

LDLs: low density lipoproteins; substances which occur in the blood and which cause infarction and other circulatory diseases.

Leucine: one of the three branched-chain amino acids.

Lipolysis: process by which one complex lipid molecule breaks down to form small elementary molecules.

Liposynthesis: process by which new fat molecules are synthesized from small simple elements.

Low carbohydrate diet: diet poor in carbohydrates, glucides.

Low fat diet: diet providing little fat.

Maltodextrins: carbohydrates made up of various linked glucose molecules.

Mitochondrion: a structure within the cytoplasm of plant and animal cells where combustion takes place to provide energy for the cell's activities; as a matter of fact, all the biochemical reactions producing aerobic energy, that is involving oxygen, occur in the mitochondrion.

Monosaccharides: simple carbohydrates consisting of one elementary molecule, like glucose or fructose.

Muesli: mixed cereals added with raisins, hazel nuts, dried apple and sometimes other dried fruits or nuts.

Oligoelements: minerals occurring in very small percentages in the human body; they include: fluorine, zinc, copper, cobalt.

One-course meal: meal consisting of either one first course or one main course - more generous portions than usual are generally allowed - preceded or followed by one dish of fresh or cooked vegetables.

pH: a measure of acidity or alkalinity of a substance; when the pH is 7 the fluid is neutral; when it is lower than 7 the fluid is acid and when it is higher than 7 the fluid is alkaline.

Plasma: the fluid component of blood, that is the blood deprived of its corpuscles (red cells, white cells and platelets).

Plicometrics: method to measure the thickness of the skin folds, plicae, by means of a special instrument: plicometer. By measuring the plicae in specific regions of the body, dietitians can easily assess the body fat concentration of a person.

Polyminerals: products containing various kinds of minerals.

Polyvitamins: products containing different kinds of vitamins.

Pre-hydration: water intake before physical exercise; pre-hydration is highly recommended in case of predictable severe sweating during the performance. It is possible to distinguish between the pre-hydration made immediately before physical practice and the pre-hydration made some time earlier - in this case, the beverage should also contain glycerin or another substance helping the body to hold water, otherwise it would be rapidly eliminated in the urine.

Re-hydration: water intake, while drinking or eating foods with a high water content, so as to re-plenish the previously lost water.

Slim down: reduce one's body fat concentration; it is important not to mistake the loss of weight, which can result from the decrease in any body component: water, muscle, glycogen..., for real slimming down.

Starch: a polysaccharide consisting of many small glucose molecules; starch occurs widely in bread, pasta, rice and potatoes, as a carbohydrate energy store.

Sucrose: common table sugar; it is a disaccharide, which means that it is made up of two linked molecules: one molecule of glucose and one of fructose.

Sugar: simple carbohydrate; however, the word 'sugar' is commonly used to refer to sucrose (table sugar).

Sweat: fluid produced by highly specialized glands: the sweat glands; the evaporation of sweat through the body surface removes heat from the body.

Sweat glands: glands producing sweat.

Synthesis: process by which new chemical compounds form from more simple compounds. In the synthesis of proteins, single amino acids link together to generate new protein molecules.

Triglycerides: very common fatty substances consisting of an ester of glycerol and three fatty acid molecules. Most of the fat occurring in adipocytes is made up of triglycerides. Triglycerides widely occur in butter and oils.

Valine: one of the three branched-chain amino acids.

Coaching Books from REEDSWAIN

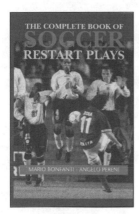

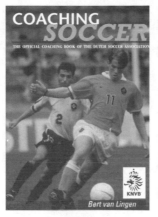

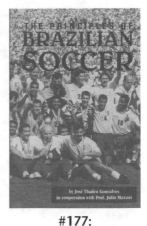

#785:
Complete Books of
Soccer Restart Plays
by Mario Bonfanti and
Angelo Pereni
$14.95

#154:
Coaching Soccer
by Bert van Lingen
$14.95

#177:
PRINCIPLES OF
Brazilian Soccer
by José Thadeu
Goncalves
in cooperation with Prof. Julio Mazzei
$16.95

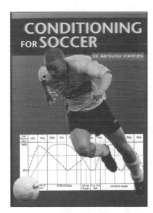

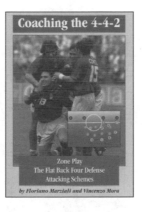

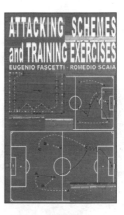

#185:
Conditioning
for Soccer
Dr. Raymond Verheijen
$19.95

#244:
Coaching the 4-4-2
by Maziali and Mora
$14.95

#765:
Attacking Schemes
and Training
Exercises
by Eugenio Fascetti and
Romedio Scaia
$14.95

Call REEDSWAIN 1-800-331-5191

Coaching Books from REEDSWAIN

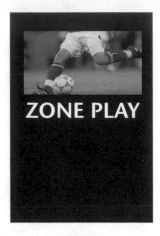

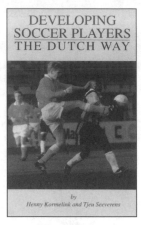

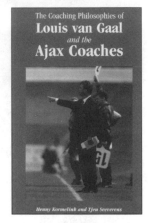

#788:
ZONE PLAY:
A Tactical and Technical
Handbook
$14.95

#267:
**Developing
Soccer Players
THE DUTCH WAY**
$12.95

#175:
The Coaching Philosophies of
Louis van Gaal
and the
Ajax Coaches
*by Kormelink and
Seeverens*

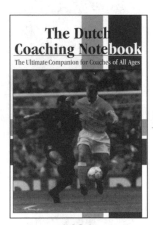

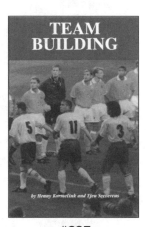

#284:
**The Dutch Coaching
Notebook**
$14.95

#287:
Team Building
by Kormelink and Seeverens
$9.95

Web Site: www.reedswain.com